OXFORD MEDICAL PUBLICATIONS

Emergencies in
Mental Health
Nursing

D1229503

Published and forthcoming titles in the Emergencies in ... series

Emergencies in Anaesthesia, Second Edition
Edited by Keith Allman, Andrew McIndoe, and Iain H. Wilson

Emergencies in Cardiology, Second Edition
Edited by Saul G. Myerson, Robin P. Choudhury, and Andrew Mitchell

Emergencies in Children's and Young People's Nursing
Edited by Edward Alan Glasper, Gillian McEwing, and Jim Richardson

Emergencies in Clinical Radiology
Edited by Richard Graham and Ferdia Gallagher

Emergencies in Clinical Surgery
Edited by Chris Callaghan, J. Andrew Bradley, and Christopher Watson

Emergencies in Critical Care
Edited by Martin Beed, Richard Sherman, and Ravi Mahajan

Emergencies in Mental Health Nursing
Edited by Patrick Callaghan and Helen Waldock

Emergencies in Nursing
Edited by Philip Downing

Emergencies in Obstetrics and Gynaecology
Edited by S. Arulkumaran

Emergencies in Oncology
Edited by Martin Scott-Brown, Roy A.J. Spence, and Patrick G. Johnston

Emergencies in Paediatrics and Neonatology
Edited by Stuart Crisp and Jo Rainbow

Emergencies in Palliative and Supportive Care
Edited by David Currow and Katherine Clark

Emergencies in Primary Care
Chantal Simon, Karen O'Reilly, John Buckmaster, and Robin Proctor

Emergencies in Psychiatry
Basant K. Puri and Ian H. Treasaden

Emergencies in Respiratory Medicine
Edited by Robert Parker, Catherine Thomas, and Lesley Bennett

Emergencies in Sports Medicine
Edited by Julian Redhead and Jonathan Gordon

Emergencies in Trauma
Aneel Bhangu, Caroline Lee, and Keith Porter

Head, Neck and Dental Emergencies
Edited by Mike Perry

Medical Emergencies in Dentistry
Nigel Robb and Jason Leitch

616.89
Em32c

Emergencies in Mental Health Nursing

Edited by

Patrick Callaghan

Professor of Mental Health Nursing,
University of Nottingham

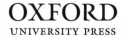

OXFORD
UNIVERSITY PRESS

3/13   EP   42.95

OXFORD
UNIVERSITY PRESS

Great Clarendon Street, Oxford OX2 6DP
United Kingdom

Oxford University Press is a department of the University of Oxford.
It furthers the University's objective of excellence in research, scholarship,
and education by publishing worldwide. Oxford is a registered trade mark of
Oxford University Press in the UK and in certain other countries

© Oxford University Press 2012

The moral rights of the authors have been asserted

First Edition published in 2012

Impression: 1

All rights reserved. No part of this publication may be reproduced, stored in
a retrieval system, or transmitted, in any form or by any means, without the
prior permission in writing of Oxford University Press, or as expressly permitted
by law, by licence or under terms agreed with the appropriate reprographics
rights organization. Enquiries concerning reproduction outside the scope of the
above should be sent to the Rights Department, Oxford University Press, at the
address above

You must not circulate this work in any other form
and you must impose this same condition on any acquirer

British Library Cataloguing in Publication Data
Data available

Library of Congress Cataloguing in Publication Data
Data available

ISBN 978–0–19–956141–4

Printed in China
by C&C Offset Printing Co. Ltd

Oxford University Press makes no representation, express or implied, that the
drug dosages in this book are correct. Readers must therefore always check
the product information and clinical procedures with the most up-to-date
published product information and data sheets provided by the manufacturers
and the most recent codes of conduct and safety regulations. The authors and
the publishers do not accept responsibility or legal liability for any errors in the
text or for the misuse or misapplication of material in this work. Except where
otherwise stated, drug dosages and recommendations are for the non-pregnant
adult who is not breast-feeding

Links to third party websites are provided by Oxford in good faith and
for information only. Oxford disclaims any responsibility for the materials
contained in any third party website referenced in this work.

Preface

At present there are no published books that are focused solely on handling emergencies in mental health nursing, yet mental health nurses are often confronted by these situations. It is intended that the book will be a useful addition to the *Emergencies in* series and will complement the *Oxford Handbook of Mental Health Nursing*. There will be some, albeit minimal, overlap with the previous book as the policy context is the same and part of the nature of mental health nursing is attempting to prevent emergencies and crisis situations happening.

What constitutes a mental health nursing emergency? It is hard to be definitive, but we have taken a pragmatic approach here. An emergency situation is one that presents a series of challenges to the nurse. These situations are challenging when they are intense, frequent, or last long enough to threaten the quality of life and/or the physical safety of people and lead to aversive or restrictive responses or exclusion from services. Such situations include being exposed to threats or actual acts of violence and aggression; in 2009/10 there were 56,718 violent assaults against staff in the NHS, of which 69% were assaults against staff in mental health settings. Other emergency situations include acts of self-injury from service users which occurs at a rate of up to 12% and patients in acute mental health wards using non-prescribed substances—figures of around 36% are common.

In this book we have included examples of how to deal with such emergency situations, the legal frameworks that may be drawn upon to handle such situations, risk assessment and management as well as considering emergencies associated with particular groups such as older adults, children and adolescents.

In line with the style of the Oxford Handbook series, we have focussed on providing the salient features of each topic and a step-by-step guide on how to care for people whose behaviour is so challenging as to constitute an emergency or crisis situation. This book is designed to be a handy, easy-to-carry text that mental health nurses can browse easily to access up-to-date, evidence-based information on handling emergencies. Each chapter is written by a specialist in their field of practice. Some further references are included at the end of each chapter should the reader wish to explore the topic in greater detail. We hope you find the book informative and a useful aid to your practice.

Patrick Callaghan
April 2010

Contents

Contributors

Dr Martin Anderson
Formerly of University of
Nottingham
School of Nursing, Midwifery &
Physiotherapy, UK

Mrs Joan Burgess
Principal Lecturer
University of Winchester
Winchester, UK

Matthew Corrigan
RMN, Child and Adolescent
Mental Health Services,
Nottinghamshire
Healthcare NHS Trust, UK

Alan Davies
Specialist Mental Health Worker,
Child and Adolescent Mental
Health Services Nottinghamshire
Healthcare NHS Trust
Nottingham, UK

Mr Guy Davis
Associate Director of Mental
Health Law
East London NHS Foundation
Trust
London, UK

Dr Tom Dening
Consultant Psychiatrist & Medical
Director
Cambridgeshire & Peterborough
NHS Foundation Trust
Fulbourn Hospital
Cambridge, UK

Zoe Hoyle
Staff Nurse, Child and Adolescent
Mental Health Services,
Nottinghamshire Healthcare NHS
Trust, UK

Phil Machin
Clinical Nurse Specialist,
Head 2 Head, Child and
Adolescent Mental Health
Services, Nottinghamshire
Healthcare NHS Trust, UK

David Manley
Nurse Consultant
Nottinghamshire Healthcare NHS
Trust, UK

Patricia McBride
Lecturer in Mental Health, School
of Health, Nursing & Midwifery,
University of the West of
Scotland, UK

Dr Jane McGregor
University of Nottingham
School of Nursing, Midwifery &
Physiotherapy, UK

Charlotte Proctor
Clinical Nurse Specialist / Acting
Ward Manager
Thorneywood Adolescent Unit
Nottinghamshire Healthcare NHS
Trust, UK

Dr Pranathi Ramachandra
Consultant Psychiatrist
Cambridge Older People's Mental
Health Services
Cambridgeshire and Peterborough
NHS Foundation Trust, UK

Sandy Redgate
Nurse Specialist Nottinghamshire
Healthcare NHS Trust, UK

Liz Tatham
Clinical Nurse Specialist and
Family Therapist, Child and
Adolescent Mental Health
Services, Nottinghamshire
Healthcare NHS Trust, UK

Mrs Johanna Turner
Clinical Nurse Specialist in Mental Health Law
East London NHS Foundation Trust
London, UK

Prof Richard Whittington
Health & Community Care Research Unit (HaCCRU)
Institute of Psychology, Health and Society
University of Liverpool
Liverpool, UK

Michael Woods
Community Psychiatric Nurse, Child and Adolescent Mental Health Services, Nottinghamshire Healthcare NHS Trust, UK

Symbols and abbreviations

📖	cross-reference
🖱	website
A&E	Accident and Emergency
ABC	airway, breathing, and circulation
ACE	angiotensin-converting enzyme
ADHD	attention deficit hyperactivity disorder
AMHP	Approved Mental Health Professional
AS	Asperger's syndrome
BNF	*British National Formulary*
CAMHS	Child and Adolescent Mental Health Services
CD	controlled drug
CPA	care programme approach
CPK	creatine phosphokinase
CTO	Community Treatment Order
CVA	cerebrovascular accident
DKA	diabetic ketoacidosis
DNR	Do Not Resuscitate
DoLS	Deprivation of Liberty Safeguards
DTs	Delirium tremens
ECG	electrocardiogram
ECT	electroconvulsive therapy
EEG	electroencephalogram
FBC	full blood count
GCS	Glasgow Coma Scale
GP	general practitioner
h	hour/s
HIV	human immunodeficiency virus
IBB	Independent Barring Board
IM	intramuscular
IV	intravenous
LBD	Lewy body/Parkinson's disease dementia
LFT	liver function test
LPA	Lasting Power of Attorney
MCA	Mental Capacity Act
MCV	mean corpuscular volume
MHA	Mental Health Act

MHRT	Mental Health Review Tribunal
MHT	Mental Health Tribunal
MI	myocardial infarction
min	minute/s
MWC	Mental Welfare Commission
NICE	National Institute for Health and Clinical Excellence
NMC	Nursing and Midwifery Council
NMS	neuroleptic malignant syndrome
NPSA	National Patient Safety Agency
NSAID	non-steroidal anti-inflammatory drug
PPE	personal protection equipment
PO	per os (orally)
NSF	National Service Framework
PEP	post-exposure prophylaxis
PRN	pro re nata (as needed)
RAP	Regulated activity provider
RMO	Responsible Medical Officer
RT	rapid tranquillization
SNRI	serotonin noradrenaline reuptake inhibitor
SSRI	selective serotonin reuptake inhibitor
SVGA	Safeguarding Vulnerable Groups Act
TCA	tricyclic antidepressant
TDM	therapeutic drug monitoring
TFT	thyroid function test
U&E	urea and electrolyte

Introduction

The care programme approach

The care programme approach (CPA), introduced in 1991, drives the planning and delivery of mental health care in the UK. It is a 'whole systems' (integrated health and social care) approach to clinical effectiveness. It is the process for managing complex and serious cases as defined in Refocusing the Care Programme Approach (Department of Health 2008). Multidisciplinary team working is fundamental to the CPA process which focuses on delivering a service with the individual using the services at its heart. The CPA aims to ensure that the following points of good practice in mental health are adhered to:

- Arrangements for assessing the health and social care needs of people in mental health services are systematic; including a mental state and risk assessment, a carer's assessment, and a vulnerable children's assessment where applicable.
- A care plan is formulated with the service user; health and social care needs and action to be taken by the services are identified, clarified, and recorded. Where a need is identified and there is no service provision available, this is recorded on an unmet needs register.
- A care coordinator (a qualified mental health professional) is appointed to keep in close touch with the service user, and to monitor their care plan.
- There are regular reviews of the care plan involving the service user and all agencies involved.

Characteristics to consider when deciding if CPA support is needed

- Severe mental disorder (including personality disorder) with high degree of clinical complexity.
- Current or potential risk(s), including:
  - Suicide, self-harm, harm to others (including history of offending).
  - Relapse history requiring urgent response.
- Self-neglect/non-concordance with treatment plan.
- Vulnerable adult; adult/child protection.
- Exploitation, e.g. financial/sexual, financial difficulties related to mental illness, disinhibition, physical/emotional abuse, cognitive impairment.
- Current or significant history of severe distress/instability or disengagement.
- Presence of non-physical comorbidity, e.g. substance misuse learning disability.
- Multiple service provision from different agencies, including: housing, physical care, employment, criminal justice, voluntary agencies.
- Currently/recently detained under Mental Health Act or referred to crisis/home treatment team.
- Significant reliance on carer(s) or has own significant caring responsibilities.

Contingency planning

The purpose of this is to prevent circumstances escalating into a crisis by detailing the arrangements to be used at short notice in circumstances where, for example, the care coordinator is not available. The contingency plan should include the information necessary to continue implementing the care plan in an interim situation. For example, by including the telephone numbers of service providers and the names and contact details of substitutes who have agreed to provide interim support, e.g. in the event that a carer is unwell/needs to be admitted to hospital.

Crisis plans

It may be helpful here to first provide a definition of crisis before outlining the requirements of a crisis plan: crisis is the subjective experience of lack of control, helplessness, and perceived inability to cope that a person experiences when he/she is faced with a stressful event that extends beyond their current repertoire of coping mechanisms.

The crisis plan is an explicit plan of action for implementation in a crisis or developing crisis situation. The crisis plan is an integral part of the care plan that specifies action to be taken in a crisis. This may include a number of factors, which come together and may place the service user and/or others at risk, e.g. becoming homeless, or may be an agreed plan of action in response to a known relapse indicator.

Crisis situations often occur out of hours and can result in emergency intervention being applied. The benefit of anticipation of the nature of a crisis is to ensure that appropriate action is taken.

Crisis plans must set out the action to be taken, based upon previous experience, if the service user is very ill, or their mental health is rapidly deteriorating. If there is disagreement about the nature of the crisis the reasons for the disagreement should be recorded.

Crisis plans, as a minimum, should ensure that all service users know how to contact the service out of hours by recording:

- Early warning and relapse indicators.
- Who the service user is most responsive to or who would like to be contacted.
- How to contact that person.
- Previous strategies which have been successful in improving responses or getting agreement for changed care/treatment, e.g. leaving them alone, calling the police, asking a carer to leave the home for a while, etc.
- Out-of-hours contact details.

Further reading

Department of Health (2003). *The care programme approach for mental health service users.*
Department of Health (2008). *Making the CPA work for you.*
Both documents are available in PDF format on the Department of Health (UK) website at
 ஃ http://www.dh.gov.uk.

Crisis intervention

Many people with severe mental health problems, such as schizophrenia and bipolar affective disorder, enjoy long periods of relative well-being punctuated by episodes of acute illness. Acute episodes, or crises, can be triggered by a variety of factors, including environmental stressors.

Whilst people experience crises in individual ways, many will feel themselves overwhelmed and no longer able to cope. They may feel hopeless, have distressing thoughts or perceptual disturbances, and be unable to engage in everyday activities. People in crisis may also have thoughts of harming themselves or others, and be at risk of acting on these thoughts.

Interventions and services

Traditionally, mental health crises have been seen as problems to be managed within the hospital environment, often through the use of physical interventions including medication. However, alternatives to psychiatric hospital care have existed for many years. For example, in the UK, the Arbours Association has over three decades of experience in running a crisis centre for people in acute distress (🕮 http://www.arbourscentre.org.uk). The development of user-led crisis services has also been supported by a leading charity, the Mental Health Foundation (🕮 http://www.mentalhealth.org.uk).

In recent years, mainstream alternatives to hospital care have started to emerge, following the principle of providing services in the least restrictive environment. In the UK, new multidisciplinary crisis intervention and home treatment teams have appeared. These aim to provide intensive, round-the-clock services, including therapeutic psychosocial interventions, rapid prescription and administration of medication, risk assessment and management, and help with practical activities. A systematic review of the effectiveness of services of this type found that:

> 'Home care crisis treatment, coupled with an ongoing home care package, is a viable and acceptable way of treating people with serious mental illnesses. If this approach is to be widely implemented, it would seem that more evaluative studies are needed.'

Good practice with people known to be vulnerable to crises includes the identification of early warning signs, and the construction of crisis management plans. These plans set out the actions to be taken in the event of acute episodes of ill health. Both should be negotiated between practitioners, service users, and their carers.

Crisis resolution services offer flexible, home-based care, 24 hours a day, 7 days a week in which service users can expect:

- Interventions to be intensive and short term (often just 2 or 3 weeks).
- A rapid response—in city areas staff should be available within the hour.
- Frequent daily visits as needed to the service user and their family or carer.

- Medication prescribing and monitoring.
- Social issues, like debt and housing, to be addressed as part of the overall care plan.
- Support and education to be available to family and carers.
- The service to determine when an individual does or does not need to go into hospital.
- Involvement to continue until the crisis is resolved.
- For the service user to be referred on to other relevant services.

Further reading

Department of Health (2001). *The mental health policy implementation guide*. London: Department of Health.

Joy, C.B., Adams, C.E., and Rice, K. (2005). Crisis intervention for people with severe mental illnesses. *Cochrane Database of Systematic Reviews*, **4**: CD001087.

Mental health assessment

Assessment is an important stage in the nursing care of people with mental health problems. It involves collecting information and using it to decide on the need for, and the nature of, any subsequent mental health care. Assessing people's mental state involves judging their psychological health; this requires experience, a degree of intelligence, self-insight, social skills, objectivity, and the ability to deal with cognitive complexities.

In an emergency situation, note:

- Appearance: simply note the patient's physical presentation—clothing, hygiene, and cultural appropriateness.
- Behaviour: briefly describe the patient's behavioural style, including agitation, retardation, and any inappropriate or unusual behaviour.
- Conversation: describe both the content of conversation, perhaps with some quotes, as well as the form, which includes the rate of conversation, as well as the logic, or otherwise, of thought processes.
- Affect and mood: note the individual's mood level, variability, range, intensity, and appropriateness.
- Perceptual abnormalities: note any psychotic symptoms, or other perceptual abnormalities, including hallucinations and delusions. These perceptual abnormalities can occur in any of the five senses.
- Cognition: describe orientation, memory, and attention, or ability to concentrate.
- Dangerousness: comment on any suicidal or homicidal ideas, beliefs, or feelings (see 📖 Chapter 3, p. 35).
- Insight: assess the patient's insight into his or her condition. This may be hard to judge, but is particularly important because of the management implications of poor treatment compliance.
- Judgement: assess the patient's level of judgement, in particular regarding safety issues. Does the patient feel that they are in control of themselves?
- Rapport: briefly comment on how you believe the interaction was between yourself and the patient, and in particular how the patient made you feel.

Personal risk factors can include:

- Hopelessness, despair, agitation, shame, guilt, anger
- Psychosis, psychotic thought processes
- Recent interpersonal crisis, especially rejection, humiliation
- Recent suicide attempt
- Recent major loss or trauma or anniversary
- Alcohol intoxication
- Drug withdrawal state
- Chronic pain or illness
- Financial difficulties, unemployment
- Impending legal prosecution or child custody issues
- Cultural or religious conflicts
- Lack of a social support network
- Unwillingness to accept help
- Difficulty accessing help due to language barriers, lack of information, lack of support, or negative experiences with mental health services.

Protective factors

Factors that may protect a person from further deterioration also need to be identified; these include:

- Strong perceived social supports
- Family cohesion
- Peer-group affiliation
- Good coping and problem-solving skills
- Positive values and beliefs.

Formulation of a plan

This would be done in consultation with colleagues where possible. Consideration needs to be given to

- The acuteness of the symptomatology
- The level of risk being presented
- The balance between the risk and protective factors
- The individual's past history, e.g. risk factors, what has helped in the past, level of insight into the current situation.

Living wills

A living will, sometimes referred to as a healthcare directive or advance directive, is a legal document drawn up by an individual who wishes to dictate how they want to be treated in hospital if they ever lose the mental capacity to be consulted. Without such an advance decision, patients deemed unable to state their views have these decisions made for them by the multidisciplinary team acting in their best interests.

Living wills and mental capacity

People can still make a living will if they are diagnosed with a mental illness, as long as they can show that they understand the implications of what they are doing. They need to be competent to make the decision in question, not necessarily to make other decisions.

Capacity or competence

Capacity or competence can be defined as the ability to understand the implications of a decision. A person is deemed to have capacity or competence if he or she:

- Can understand and retain information relevant to the decision in question (the definition of 'to retain information' has to be assessed on an individual basis).
- Believes it, and can reflect on that information to arrive at a choice and use that information as part of the decision-making process.
- Can then express or otherwise communicate that choice.

Advantages

Creating a living will or advance directive can bring some reassurance to a person worried about their future healthcare. When healthcare professionals are faced with difficult decisions about what treatment or care to give, a living will can provide the best possible guide, and will help to ensure that the person's wishes are taken into account.

Preparing a living will can open up a dialogue with care coordinators and the multidisciplinary team that fits very neatly with the CPA and crisis planning. The process can also stimulate conversation with family and close friends, relieving them of some of the burden of decision-making at what can be a distressing time.

The British Medical Association supports the principle of advance decisions, and recognizes that healthcare professionals may be legally liable if they disregard the contents of a valid advance decision.

Are advance decisions legally enforceable?

As long as an advance decision is valid and applicable, it is legally enforceable in England and Wales:

- *Valid:* the person who drew up the advance decision must have had mental capacity to do so at the time.
- *Applicable:* the wording of the advance decision has to be relevant to the medical circumstances. If the wording is vague or there is a concern that the person was not referring to medical conditions and/ or practices that they are actually experiencing, then the advance decision may not influence the doctors' decisions at all.

The advance decision must also:
- Be clear and unambiguous.
- Have been written when the person had sufficient mental capacity.
- Have been written after the person was fully informed about the consequences of refusal of treatment, including the fact that it may hasten death.
- Have been intended to apply in the situation which has arisen.
- Not have been drawn up under the influence of other people.

What an advance decision cannot do

An advance decision cannot be used to:
- Refuse basic nursing care essential to keep a person safe and comfortable, such as washing or close observations.
- Refuse the offer of food or drink by mouth.
- Refuse the use of measures solely designed to maintain comfort, e.g. painkillers.
- Demand treatment that a healthcare team considers inappropriate.
- Ask for anything that is against the law, such as euthanasia or assisting someone in taking their own life.

The use of living wills in mental healthcare is rare although not unheard of. As part of crisis and contingency planning individuals have the opportunity to stipulate what they want to happen at this time. Living wills have been used for patients who do not wish to be resuscitated and to stipulate their care environment, e.g. a women-only ward and not in a mixed intensive care unit.

Looking after yourself

As a nurse you have a duty to yourself and your patients to act promptly if you feel that there are early warning signs that your mental health may be affecting your performance. It is recognized that mental health nursing can be demanding and stressful.

The psychiatric morbidity survey of adults (2007) (McManus et al. 2009) living in private households found that 1 in 6 (16.2%) of the adult population surveyed in England exhibited symptoms in the week prior to interview sufficient to warrant a diagnosis of a common mental health problem. This indicates that 1 in 6 of the multidisciplinary team may be experiencing a mental health problem at any given time.

Be aware of:
- Difficulties sleeping
- Becoming more impatient or irritable
- Difficulties in concentrating
- Being unable to make decisions
- Drinking or smoking too much
- Not enjoying food as much
- Increased anxiety
- Being unable to relax
- Feeling tense
- Somatic symptoms, e.g. recurrent headache, frequent colds, general aches and pains.

Take positive action
- Eat regular, healthy meals. Cut down on, or avoid, alcohol, and sugary foods, and remember to eat your 5 portions of fruit and vegetables a day.
- Taking regular exercise can improve your mood, help you to relax, and give you more energy.
- Make time for hobbies, doing the things you enjoy and spending time with friends.
- Don't make unreasonable demands on yourself or push yourself too hard. Value yourself and all that you have to offer.
- Try to talk to people you trust, your friends and family, about worries or problems. Don't be afraid to ask for help and support when you need it.
- Don't hate yourself for being who you are.
- Don't judge yourself harshly.
- Set yourself achievable goals and standards—reward yourself if you achieve these, and don't punish yourself if you do not.

If you are concerned or worried about your own mental well-being there are a number of options:
- You can talk to NHS Direct on 0845 46 47 or visit ♫ http://www. nhsdirect.nhs.uk.
- You can talk to your general practitioner (GP) or other health worker—they can help you to decide what level of support you need and refer you to other agencies if appropriate.

- You can also talk to your occupational health service at your place of work.
- Most Trusts have a confidential staff counselling service that accepts self-referrals.

Manage risk

You must act without delay if you believe that you, a colleague, or anyone else may be putting someone at risk.

Further reading

McManus, S., Meltzer, H., Brugha, T., *et al.* (Eds.) (2009). Adult psychiatric morbidity in England, 2007. Results of a household survey. Leeds: The NHS Information Centre for Health and Social Care.

Nursing and Midwifery Council (2008). *The code: standards of conduct, performance and ethics for nurses and midwives*. Available at: http://www.nmc-uk.org/Nurses-and-midwives/The-code/The-code-in-full/.

Violence and aggression

❶ Managing risk: overview

The ABC of functional assessment (analysis)
- Antecedents: what situation provokes the behaviour?
- Behaviour: what is the behavioural response to the antecedents?
- Consequences: what are the consequences of the behavioural response?

Formulating the problem
- How serious is the risk?
- Is the risk specific or general?
- How immediate is the risk?
- How volatile is the risk?
- Are circumstances likely to arise that will increase risk?
- What specific treatment and management plan can best reduce risk?

❶ Risk assessment: violence

Introduction
Risk is the likelihood of behaviour that may be harmful or beneficial for self or others. Risk assessment involves analysing potential outcomes of this behaviour; risk management involves devising a care plan to minimize harmful behaviour and maximize beneficial behaviour.

Prevalence of violence in the UK
- 65,000 violent incidents in the NHS in 2009/10.
- Mental health and learning disability settings accounted for 38,959 of these incidents.
- There were 192 assaults per 1000 staff in mental health and learning disability settings.

Consequences of violence
- Sickness from work
- Physical injury, sometimes serious
- Post-traumatic stress disorder
- Malignant alienation
- Persistent fear.

Demographic predictors of violence
- Previous history of violence to people or property
- History of misuse of substances or alcohol
- Previous expression of intent to harm others
- Evidence of rootlessness or social restlessness
- Previous dangerous/impulsive acts
- Previous use of weapons
- Denial of previous established dangerous acts
- Verbal threats of violence.

Clinical predictors of violence
- Misuse of drugs or alcohol
- Drug effects (e.g. disinhibition)
- Delusions or hallucinations focused on a particular person
- Command hallucinations
- Preoccupation with violent fantasy
- Delusions of control
- Agitation, excitement, overt hostility or suspiciousness
- Poor collaboration with suggested treatments
- Organic dysfunction.

Situational predictors of violence

- Extent of social support
- Immediate availability of potential weapon
- Relationship to victim
- Access to potential victim
- Limit setting
- Staff attitudes.

Antecedents and warning signs

- Tense and angry facial expressions
- Increased or prolonged restlessness
- General overarousal of systems
- Increased volume of speech, erratic movements
- Prolonged eye contact
- Discontentment, refusal to communicate, withdrawal, fear, irritation
- Unclear thought processes, poor concentration
- Delusions or hallucinations with violent content
- Verbal threats or gestures
- Reporting anger or violent feelings
- Replicating previous behaviour that led to violence.

Risk assessment

- Regular and comprehensive assessment
- Assessment of staff attitudes, situations, organizational and environmental factors linked to violence
- A structured and sensitive interview with user to focus on triggers, early warning signs, and other vulnerabilities
- Avoid negative assumptions based on ethnicity
- Multidisciplinary approach
- Assess and record users' preferences for managing violence.

Actuarial measures that can be used in risk assessment

The Historical/Clinical/Risk Management 20 (HCR-20) uses 20 items in relation to the assessment and management of individuals who are potentially violent: 10 historical items, 5 clinical items, and 5 risk management items (see Table 2.1). It is free to use from ᗆ http://www.scotland.gov.uk/maclean/docs/svso-23.asp

Other measures that may be appropriate, but which have usage costs, are:

- Psychopathy checklist (PCL-R)
- Violence Risk Appraisal Guide (VRAG)
- Dangerous Behaviour Rating Scale (DBRS).

Table 2.1 HCR-20 assessment tool items

Subscales	Items
Historical scale	
H1	Previous violence
H2	Young age at first violent incident
H3	Relationship instability
H4	Employment problems
H5	Substance use problems
H6	Major mental illness
H7	Psychopathy
H8	Early maladjustment
H9	Personality disorder
H10	Prior supervision failure
Clinical scale	
C1	Lack of insight
C2	Negative attitudes
C3	Active symptoms of major mental illness
C4	Impulsivity
C5	Unresponsive to treatment
Risk management scale	
R1	Plans lack feasibility
R2	Exposure to destabilizers
R3	Lack of personal support
R4	Non-compliance with remediation attempts
R5	Stress

Further reading

Morgan, S. (2000). *Clinical Risk Management: A Clinical Tool and Practitioner Manual.* London: The Sainsbury Centre for Mental Health.

National Institute for Health and Clinical Excellence (2005). *Violence: The Short Term management of disturbed/violent behaviour in psychiatric in-patient settings and emergency departments* (Clinical Guideline 25), London: NICE. Available at: ℛ http://guidance.nice.org.uk/CG25

Yang, M., Wong, C.P., & Coid, J. (2010). The Efficacy iof Violence Risk Prediction: A Meta-Analytic Comparison of Nie Risk Assessment Tools. *Psychological Bulletin* **136**(5):740-767.

❶ Risk assessment: abuse

Introduction

Risk is the likelihood of behaviour that may be harmful or beneficial for self or others. Risk assessment involves analysing potential outcomes of this behaviour; risk management involves devising a care plan to minimize harmful behaviour and maximize beneficial behaviour.

Types of abuse

- Physical: punching, pushing, hitting.
- Sexual: rape, sexual assault, sexual acts without consent or where consent could not be given.
- Psychological: emotional abuse, threats, humiliation.
- Financial: theft, fraud, exploitation.
- Neglect: ignoring needs, withholding necessities of life.
- Discrimination: racism, sexism, ageism, harassment (bullying).
- Institutional: poor professional service, ill treatment.

Risk factors associated with abuse

- All: unequal power, social isolation, vulnerable family history of violence and abuse.
- Physical: long delays in reporting injuries, unexplained bruises, misuse of medication.
- Sexual: overly sexual conversations and behaviour.
- Psychological: ambivalence about carer, unexplained paranoia, passivity/resignation.
- Financial: unusual account activity, excessive gifts to carers.
- Neglect: person left alone in unsafe environment, refusal of access to visitors/callers, violating privacy and dignity.
- Rights violation: coercion, refusal of access to visitors/callers, lack of respect, lack of attention to personal hygiene.
- Institutional: rigid routines, poor standards of cleanliness, 'batch' care, i.e. care that is not individualized.

Risk assessment

- Conduct assessment interview.
- Mental state assessment.
- Take history of abuse incidents.
- Assess specific indicators of abuse (see 📖 Risk factors associated with abuse, p. 20).
- Assess for any discrepancies between what is reported and what is observed.
- Assess for any discrepancies between verbal and non-verbal cues.
- Assess coping potential and availability of social support.

Assessing the seriousness of abuse
- Vulnerability of individual.
- Nature and extent of abuse.
- Length of time of abuse.
- Impact on individual.
- Repeated or increasingly serious acts of abuse.
- Intent of person alleged responsible for abuse.

Management
- Ensure safety of victim.
- Discuss concerns with colleagues/multidisciplinary team.
- Make appropriate referrals to care management team/social services team/police/registration inspection unit.
- Consider what treatment or therapy is appropriate.
- Ensure modification in the way that services are provided.
- Support individual through appropriate action he/she takes to seek justice or redress.
- Use stress management techniques.
- Encourage the vulnerable person to remain active and independent, maintaining social contacts.
- Work with significant others to discuss best forms of support/ aftercare.

Further reading
Department of Health (2000). *Domestic Violence: A resources manual for health care professionals.* London: Department of Health.

Oxleas Mental Health Trust (2002). *A Guide to the assessment and management of risk.* London: Oxleas Mental Health Trust, pp. 37–59.

❶ Risk assessment: falls

Introduction

Risk is the likelihood of behaviour that may be harmful or beneficial for self or others. Risk assessment involves analysing potential outcomes of this behaviour; risk management involves devising a care plan to minimize harmful behaviour and maximize beneficial behaviour.

Areas to cover in assessment

- Risk factors
- History
- Physical health
- Environmental factors
- Information from relatives and carers
- Ideation/mental state
- Intent
- Planning
- Person's awareness of risk
- Benefits and harm from risk
- Formulation.

Risk factors (Table 2.2)

Table 2.2 Variables and risk factors of falls

Variable	Higher risk	Lower risk
Age	Older	Younger
Past history	Incidence of falls in past 12mths	No history of falls
Physical status	Medical problems esp. circulatory	No/few medical problems
Environment	Hazardous	No hazards
Mental state	Sensory and cognitive impairment	No sensory or cognitive impairments
Medication	Combinations affecting balance	Combinations that do not affect balance
Mobility	Poor: gait/balance problems	No problems

Risk assessment

- 'SPLATT':
  - Symptoms
  - Previous falls
  - Location
  - Activity
  - Time
  - Trauma.

- Assess significant others' views.
- Ideation and mental state: awareness of illness, vulnerability, capacity to make decisions.
- Awareness of risk.
- Benefit and harm from risk.

Multifactorial falls risk assessment

- Identification of falls history.
- Assessment of gait, balance, mobility, and muscle weakness.
- Assessment of osteoporosis risk.
- Assessment of person's perceived functional ability and fear of falling.
- Assessment of visual impairment.
- Assessment of cognitive impairment and neurological examination.
- Assessment of urinary incontinence.
- Assessment of home hazards.
- Cardiovascular examination and review.

Multifactorial management

- Strength and balance training.
- Home hazard assessment and intervention.
- Vision assessment and referral for treatment if necessary.
- Medication review with modification/withdrawal.
- Cardiac pacing.
- Oral and written information to users and significant others about recommended measures to prevent further falls and how to cope with a fall.

Rating scales for assessing falls risk

- FRASE (Falls Risk Assessment for Elderly).
- STRATIFY (St Thomas Risk Assessment Tool in Falling Elderly).

Further reading

National Institute for Health and Clinical Excellence (2004). *Falls: the assessment and prevention of falls in older people* (Guideline 21). London: NICE. Available at: ℗ http://guidance.nice.org.uk/CG21

Oxleas Mental Health Trust (2002). *A Guide to the assessment and management of risk.* London: Oxleas Mental Health Trust, pp. 107–17.

❶ Risk assessment: suicide

Introduction

Risk is the likelihood of behaviour that may be harmful or beneficial for self or others. Risk Assessment involves analysing potential outcomes of this behaviour; risk management involves devising a care plan to minimize harmful behaviour and maximize beneficial behaviour.

Assessing suicide risk

- Risk factors
- History
- Information from relatives and carers
- Ideation/mental state
- Intent
- Planning
- Person's awareness of risk
- Benefits and harm from risk
- Formulation.

Predictors of suicide risk

- History of self-harm
- Loss of contact with mental health services within 1 week of discharge
- Depression
- Dual diagnosis
- Inpatient care
- Member of ethnic minority
- Homelessness.

Risk factors (Table 2.3)

See also 📖 Psychiatric emergencies, p. 84.

Table 2.3 Higher- and lower-risk factors of suicide

Higher risk	Lower risk
Males aged >65, or 15–30 years	Younger females
Separated, widowed, divorced	Married/stable relationship
Lives alone, socially isolated	Good social network
Poor physical health	Good physical health
Poor mental health	No previous episodes
Substance misuse	No substance misuse
Previous episodes of self-harm	No episodes of self-harm
Actual or attempted self-harm suicide by relative	No family history
Loss of supports	
Hopelessness, despair, loss of interest	
Mild learning disability	

Assessment of needs
- Assessment should be comprehensive.
- Include evaluation of social, psychological, and motivational factors specific to acts of self-harm, current suicidal intent, and mental and social needs assessment

Assessment of risk
- Identification of main clinical and demographic features associated with risk of further self-harm.
- Identification of key psychological characteristics associated with risk, e.g. depression, hopelessness, and continuing intent

Further reading

National Institute for Health and Clinical Excellence (2004). *Self-Harm: The short-term physical and psychological management and secondary prevention of self-harm in primary and secondary care* (Clinical Guideline 16). London: NICE. Available at: ℛ http://guidance.nice.org.uk/CG16

Semple, D., Smyth, R., Burns, J., et al. (Eds.) (2005). *Oxford Handbook of Psychiatry*. Oxford: Oxford University Press.

❶ Risk assessment: fire

Introduction

Risk is the likelihood of behaviour that may be harmful or beneficial for self or others. Risk assessment involves analysing potential outcomes of this behaviour; risk management involves devising a care plan to minimize harmful behaviour and maximize beneficial behaviour.

Areas to cover in assessment

- Risk factors
- History
- Information from relatives and carers
- Ideation/mental state
- Intent
- Planning
- Person's awareness of risk
- Benefits and harm from risk
- Formulation.

Risk factors (Table 2.4)

Table 2.4 Variables and risk factors of fires

Variable	Higher risk	Lower risk
Past history of arson	Past history, especially recent younger age at first fire setting	No history
Past history of accidental fire setting	Past history, especially recent	No history
Use of potential sources of fire	Poor safety awareness	Good safety awareness
	Smoker	Non-smoker
	Unsafe appliances	Safe appliances
	Unsafe behaviour, e.g. leaving pots unattended, leaving gas on, overloading electric circuits	Safe behaviour
Environment	Potential fuel for fire	Little potential fuel for fire
	No fire alerting system	
	Electrical cords under furniture or carpeting	Fire alerting system, e.g. working smoke alarm
Learning disability	Mild learning disability with poor social and communication skills	Severe learning disability

Risk assessment

- The person: do they exhibit risk factors? Do they exhibit safety awareness?
- The environment: is there potential fuel for fires? Is there a fire alerting system? Is there a potential fire escape and is the person able to use it?
- Other people: is there a potential risk to others?

Assessment of nature of previous fires

- Recency: how recent was the risk or behaviour?
- Severity.
- Frequency: was it an isolated incident, or does it happen more frequently?
- Pattern: is there a common pattern to the type of incident or the context in which it occurs?

Management of risk of fires

- Further specialist assessment.
- Admission to hospital if arson intent is present.
- Make the person's environment safer.
- Provision of fire alerting devices.
- Supervision during procedures that may be risky, e.g. cooking, smoking, using appliances.

Further reading

Oxleas Mental Health Trust (2002). *A guide to the assessment and management of risk.* London: Oxleas Mental Health Trust, pp. 119–30.

❶ Risk assessment: self-neglect

Introduction

Risk is the likelihood of behaviour that may be harmful or beneficial for self or others. Risk assessment involves analysing potential outcomes of this behaviour; risk management involves devising a care plan to minimize harmful behaviour and maximize beneficial behaviour.

Areas to cover in assessment for self-neglect

- Hygiene
- Diet
- Physical health
- Medication
- Substance misuse
- Adequacy of clothing
- Capacity to self-care
- Capacity to seek help
- Adequacy accommodation
- Household safety
- Basic household amenities
- Infestation
- Financial situation.

Risk factors linked to self-neglect (Table 2.5)

See also 📖 Psychiatric emergencies, p. 84.

Table 2.5 Higher- and lower-risk factors linked to self-neglect

Higher risk	Lower risk
Female	Male
Living alone	Living with others
Mental illness; dementia, psychosis	No mental illness
Single, widowed, separated	Married/stable relationship
Substance misuse	No substance misuse
Poor housing	Good accommodation
Loss of significant other	No loss of significant other
Poor physical health	Good health
Sensory or cognitive impairments	No sensory or cognitive impairments
Unable to seek help	Able to seek help
Vulnerable to exploitation	Living with competent carers

Risk assessment

- History: awareness of illness/vulnerability, capacity to identify, understand, and manage risks, engagement with treatment, aftercare services, premorbid personality.
- View of significant others: expressions of concerns.
- Ideation and mental state: capacity to make decisions and think about ways to manage risks, willingness to accept support, present state examination.
- Intent: degree of intent to engage in a risky behaviour.
- Planning: assess whether the person has made any plans to engage in risky behaviour.
- Awareness of risk: assessment of the person's view of problem.
- Benefit and harm of risk: assessment of the benefits versus the harm of risky behaviour. What is risky behaviour in respect of neglect?—little in the way of behaviour in relation to the above table as these are more problems related to people than them engaging in risky behaviour. Risky behaviour includes: unhealthy diet, using illegal substances, poor self-hygiene, and using medications differently for what they were prescribed.

Management

- CPA is important in this respect.
- Plan care with user and significant others.
- Identify antecedents of self-neglect behaviour (covered earlier in this topic).
- Increased monitoring.
- Access to supported housing.
- Use of Section 117 ('Aftercare and the Care Programme Approach' of the Mental Health Act) if necessary.
- Environmental Health assessment and treatment of property if necessary.

Further reading

Johnson, J. and Adams, J. (1996). Self-neglect in later life. *Health and Social Care in the Community* **4**(4): 226–33.

Oxleas Mental Health Trust (2002). *A guide to the assessment and management of risk*. London: Oxleas Mental Health Trust, pp. 23–35.

❶ Challenging behaviours

Definition of challenging behaviour

Challenging behaviour is an action outside cultural norms of such intensity, duration, or frequency that it jeopardizes the safety of the person or others, and may restrict the person's access to services.

Examples of challenging behaviour

- Violence
- Self-injury
- Total compliance
- Ambivalence
- Non-compliance
- Socially unacceptable behaviour
- Sexual disinhibition
- Substance use.

Epidemiology of challenging behaviour

- 6–14% in LD (learning difficulty) settings (of the 6–14%, up to 15% is self-injury)
- 36.3% (substance misuse) in MHfacilities
- 3–12% (self-injury) among children in community
- 56,718 incidents in 2009/10 involving 1,278,071 staff, approx 44 assaults per staff.

Aetiology of challenging behaviour

- Biological factors, e.g. genetic, neurochemistry, brain structure and function
- Psychological factors, e.g. social learning
- Social factors, e.g. social control.

Why is some behaviour challenging?

- Other people will not like it and the person can be excluded from society.
- It stops people getting to know each other.
- Someone could get hurt.
- It impairs interpersonal relationships.
- It could cause damage to property.

What functions does challenging behaviour serve?

- Avoidance
- Attention
- Sensory—internally rewarding
- Tangible—externally rewarding.

Common antecedents of challenging behaviour

- Feeling bullied
- Fear
- Boredom
- Invasion of personal space
- Frustration at not being listened to
- Not being understood
- Effect of medication/drugs.

Managing challenging behaviours—general tips

- Remain calm.
- Do not make rash promises.
- Show empathy and concern.
- Treat people with respect.

What works in managing challenging behaviour?

- Functional analysis +++
- Behaviour modification +++
- Cognitive behavioural therapy +++
- De-escalation +
- Breakaway +
- Restraint ++
- Medication +.

What seems to make things worse?

- Ignoring the function of behaviour.
- Not applying long-term interventions.
- Negative staff reactions.
- Lack of involvement of staff in designing and applying behavioural programmes.
- Insufficient staff time and attention.

The ABC of functional assessment (analysis)

- Antecedents: what situation provokes the behaviour?
- Behaviour: what is the behavioural response to the antecedents?
- Consequences: what are the consequences of the behavioural response?

Summary

- People's behaviour communicates information about their thoughts, feelings, and beliefs.
- Treating people with respect and courtesy is likely to minimize your exposure to challenging behaviour.
- Analysing the function that challenging behaviour serves is crucial to managing the behaviour effectively.
- Behavioural approaches are shown to be effective at managing challenging behaviours.
- Ignoring challenging behaviour is likely to make it worse.

Further reading

Addison, M. (2000). Supporting Behaviour Change (using a Functional Assessment to understand the function of the behaviour). [Information leaflet]. University of Kent: Challenging Behaviour Foundation. Available at: ♒ http://www.thecbf.org.uk/chall-behaviour/funct-assess.htm

Emerson, E. (1995). *Challenging Behaviour. Analysis and Intervention in People with Learning Disabilities.* Cambridge: Cambridge University Press.

National Institute for Health and Clinical Excellence (2005). *Violence: The short-term management of disturbed/violent behaviour in in-patient psychiatric settings and emergency departments* (Clinical Guideline 25). London: NICE. Available at: ♒ http://guidance.nice.org.uk/CG25

Sense Scotland (2003). *Challenging our approaches to behaviour.* Edinburgh: Sense Scotland Practice Development Department.

Xenditis, K., Russell, A., and Murphy, D. (2001). Management of people with challenging behaviour. *Archives in Psychiatric Treatment* **7**: 109–16.

❶ Conflict resolution and management

What is conflict?

Conflict has been described as 'A disagreement through which the parties involved perceive a threat to their needs, interests, or concerns' (University of Wisconsin, OHRD, 2006).

The nature of conflict

- Disagreements.
- Complaints or criticism of someone's performance, behaviour, or attitude.
- Excluding or ignoring others: being silently contemptuous.
- A matching of wills.
- Deliberating opposing a request or instruction.
- Perceiving someone to be deliberately provocative.
- Taking risks and threatening the security of others.
- Aggressive behaviour.

Causes of conflict

- Emotional states
- Different opinions, beliefs, values
- Power and control
- Varying facts or data
- Alternative methods or processes
- Alternative goals.

Conflict styles and consequences

- Competing
- Accommodating
- Avoiding
- Compromising
- Collaborating.

Responses to conflict

- Emotional
- Cognitive
- Physical.

How perceptions impact upon conflict

- Culture, race, and ethnicity
- Gender and sexuality
- Knowledge of situation at hand
- Impressions of the messenger
- Previous experiences.

Resolving conflict
- Maintain contact between parties.
- Look for the needs and interests that lie behind fixed positions.
- Identify and safe place for negotiation.
- Actively listen.
- Approach problem solving with flexibility.
- Manage impasse with clam, patience, and respect.
- Build an agreement that works.

What works in resolving conflict?
- Strong social and global self-efficacy.
- Strong group identity.
- First-line management support moderates the impact of conflict.

Summary
- Understanding the nature and causes of conflict will help resolve it.
- Think about how your interaction style might contribute to conflict.
- Manage conflict in a manner that allows you to maintain a working relationship and achieve your goals.

Further reading
Desivilya, H.S. and Eizen, D. (2005). Conflict management in work teams: the role of social self-efficacy and group identification. *International Journal of Conflict Management* **16**(2): 183–208.

Heron, J. (2001). *Helping the client: A Creative Practical Guide* (5th edition). London: Sage.

Pardey, D. (2007). *Introducing Leadership*. Oxford: Butterworth-Heineman, Chapter 9, 'Handling conflict', pp. 159–70.

Thomas, J.L., Bliese, P.D., and Jex, S.M. (2005). Interpersonal conflict and organisational commitment: Examining two levels of supervisory support as multi-level moderators. *Journal of Applied Social Psychology* **35**(11): 2375–98.

University of Wisconsin Office of Human Resource Development (2006). *Conflict Resolution*. Available at: 🖱 http://www.ohrd.wisc.edu/onlinetraining/resolution/aboutwhatisit.htm

Webne-Behrman, H. (1998). *The Practice of Facilitation: Managing Group Processes and Solving Problems*. Westport, CT: Quorum Books.

Self-harm and suicidal behaviour

Introduction

Definition of self-harm

Self-harm is the term often used to refer to a range of behaviours. This usually encapsulates actions involving a form of self-injury, self-mutilation, or overdose. The act may or may not be motivated by suicidal intention. Intent can only be properly established by interviewing the service user and understanding their motivations. People who present with self-harm may clearly not wish to end their own life, but people who are suicidal may have a clear intent to take their own life. It is important to recognize 'self-harm' as a very individual act involving the experience of stress, emotional pain, and personal crisis. This understanding should be at the centre of clinical practice and at the centre of the work being negotiated and planned. The National Institute for Health and Clinical Excellence (NICE) has produced guidelines for the management and care of people who self-harm within primary and secondary care. The National Strategy for Suicide Prevention in England provides details on the key goals in suicide prevention, including work with people who have self-harmed and who have attempted suicide (see 📖 'Further reading', p. 37).

Types of self-harm

- Cutting
- Ingestion/overdose of medication
- Hand/fist banging
- Burning (cigarettes or caustic substances, often of the skin)
- Drinking noxious substances
- Scratching
- Excessive scrubbing of the skin.

Non-suicidal repetitive self-harm

- Low/no level of suicide intent/wish to die.
- May be a personal system of control.
- Person is expert in the behaviour engaged in.
- Behaviour is important to the person.
- Is not simply attention-seeking behaviour or a cry for help.
- Person always still has right to respect and dignity.

Note: the risk of suicide may increase if an attempt to remove behaviour is made.

Examples of reasons for self-harm

Self-harm is a very individual act. People will have their own reasons for self-harm and these will be complex and multifaceted. The following are examples only (see also 📖 Psychiatric emergencies, p. 84):

- Relationship problems/breakdown
- Loss separation/divorce/parental divorce
- Poor problem-solving skills
- May be part of a process of recovery
- A mechanism to help cope/resolve difficult feelings
- Trauma from past physical, sexual, or emotional abuse
- Alcohol/drug misuse (in young people)

- Alcohol/drug misuse (in adults). May also be a reason for self-harm in young people if parents/guardians are misusing alcohol/drugs
- Imprisonment/period in custody
- Difficulties in communicating/interpersonal expression
- A method of communication
- Abusive relationships
- Bullying
- Personal shame (e.g. sexuality)
- Poor social/immediate support from others
- Peer rejection
- Racism/racial abuse.

Methods of suicide (common)
- Hanging, strangulation, and suffocation
- Drug-related self-poisoning
- Motor gas poisoning
- Drowning
- Jumping/falling in front of moving object
- Jumping/falling from high places
- Use of sharp object
- Firearms and explosives
- Smoke, fire, and flames.

Further reading

Department of Health (2002). *National Suicide Prevention Strategy for England*. London: HMSO.

McLaughlin, C. (2007). *Suicide-Related Behaviour. Understanding, Caring and Therapeutic Responses*. John Wiley and Sons, Ltd, West Sussex.

National Institute for Health and Clinical Excellence (2004). *Self-Harm: The Short Term Physical and Psychological Management and Secondary Prevention if Self-Harm in Primary and Secondary Care*. Leicester and London: British Psychological Society.

❶ Assessment and risk in suicide and self-harm

Reasons for suicide

The risk factors identified in Box 3.1 are important as the evidence demonstrates that they are strongly associated reasons for suicide (see also 📖 Psychiatric emergencies, p. 84). Like self-harm, suicide is an individual act. The reasons for an attempted suicide will be personal and complex. The list given in Box 3.1 is a guide to support knowledge. It may be possible to identify many of these factors in a person but on the other hand very few or none will apply. Use the listed 'key aspects' to help in the assessment. Take note to observe for the events that may have 'tipped' the person over the edge. For example:

- Bills that cannot be paid
- Loss of work
- Argument with contractor/work
- Partner filing for divorce or leaving
- Criminal charges
- Death of a relative, friend, significant other
- Other relationship problems.

Check for:

- Combination of events
- Build up over a period of time, especially unhappy relationships
- Significant event.

Key aspects of assessment

- Ensure a full psychosocial assessment is carried out.
- Assessment is ongoing and carried out over a period of time.
- Therapeutic value to person—being able to talk.
- Will be inexact at times.
- Check for risk factors (Box 3.1).
- Focus on the person and individuality.
- Consider one's own 'gut reaction' i.e. 'This doesn't feel right'.
- Be aware of your own intuitive sense.
- Use assessment tools (see 📖 'Tests for risk of suicide', p. 44)

Use of risk factors in assessment

Risk is the probability or chance of a particular event occurring in the future. In terms of suicide risk the level of risk is referred to in terms of a sliding rule between high and low risk. Risk is dynamic and not static. It is important to note:

- Features of risk vary between groups.
- Vulnerability may fluctuate.
- Initial period of inpatient stay is an at-risk time.
- Discharge period is an at-risk time.
- During withdrawn/severe depression when a person starts to show improvement there is an increased risk of suicide.
- Observe for sudden motivation/energy.

Box 3.1 Risk factors for suicide

- Gender:
  - Being male
- Age:
  - Younger age group (19–34 years)
  - Older age group (85+ years)
- Health:
  - Physical health conditions, e.g., chronic medical illness
- Social factors:
  - Relationship problems
  - Unemployment, social deprivation, and poverty
  - Financial difficulties
  - Legal problems
  - Abuse—past, present (sexual, physical, emotional)
  - Divorced, widowed, bereavement/loss
  - Loss of valued role, e.g. retirement
  - Loss of parents through divorce or death during childhood
  - Being single
  - Living alone (also loneliness)/social isolation/social network
  - Homelessness
  - Social class (1 & 5)
  - Occupation (professional groups such as doctors)
  - Being a prisoner/in criminal justice system
  - Imitation and contagion—exposure to suicidal behaviour other/media including the Internet
- Experience of mental health issues:
  - Previous history of self-harm/suicide attempts (especially where planned delay in discovery has been evident and notes left)
  - Depression (other common mental health problems)
  - Hopelessness (especially feeling of entrapment and unable to solve problems)
  - Serious mental health problems
  - Alcohol problems and drug misuse
  - Personality disorder (comorbid with other mental health problems)
  - Family history of suicide
  - Recent contact with mental health services
- Intent:
  - High intent features
  - Choice of method—violent (hanging, jumping in front of a train, shotgun)
  - Access to means of suicide
- Plans for death (changing of will, family farewells).

Further reading

Anderson, M. and Jenkins, R. (2006). The National Suicide Prevention Strategy for England: the reality of a national strategy for the nursing profession. *Journal of Psychiatric and Mental Health Nursing* **13**: 641–50.

Hawton, K. (2005). *Prevention and Treatment of Suicidal Behaviour: From Science to Practice*. Oxford: Oxford University Press.

❶ Factors that may protect people from suicide

Protective factors—general examples

While risk factors may be evident there will also be factors that may protect against suicide:

- Restricted access to lethal means
- Effective clinical assessment and care
- Easy access to therapeutic interventions
- Support for help seeking
- Social support
- Confiding, supportive relationship.

Protective factors for young people—examples

- Good self-esteem and problem-solving skills
- Good emotional relationship with at least one person in family
- Good social support and social network
- Religious beliefs.

Protective factors for older people—examples

- Marriage (men)
- Children (women)
- Religious beliefs
- Interests/social engagement/hobby
- Good coping skills
- Social support and social interactions
- A confiding, supportive relationship.

☼ Management of suicide risk

Key actions and interventions for immediate risk of suicide

Immediate observations of 'individual factors' in the person presenting:

Check for decreases in factors such as:

- Social contact (work, family, friends)
- Pleasure
- Drive
- Tolerance
- Health
- Sleep
- Appetite.

Check for increases in factors such as:

- Irritability
- Alcohol (amount/drinking on own)
- Bills/debts
- Avoidance
- Being on own
- Feeling useless
- No hope
- Unfinished things
- Losses.

Check the duration and context of the change/s

- Has it been rapid?
- Is what was down now suddenly now ok?
- High alcohol intake
- Has the drinking now suddenly stopped?
- Bad reaction to a loss
- Feeling of no future
- What is particularly different?

Check what is being revealed when person is talking

- Suicidal ideas
- Previous attempts of suicide
- Relationship issues
- Mental health problems
- Financial/work/study/health issues
- Substance misuse.

❶ Assessing risk in special settings

Acute suicide risk (inpatient settings)

- The priority is to establish and maintain a therapeutic relationship (based on interpersonal skills/interventions outlined below). These skills need to be implemented at all times including during formal observations if they are used.
- Check individual status against legal powers i.e. Mental Health Act, common law.
- Implement appropriate level of observation (high, medium, low).

High: observe the person at all times

- Restrict person to unit environment.
- Remove all potentially harmful objects and substances.
- Identify any possible ligature points.

Note: ligature points should be globally assessed within the clinical environment on a yearly basis; however, on occasion where a service user is very determined and desperate it is possible for them to fashion ligature points in unexpected places. It is therefore worth taking extra care to observe the environment, including bathrooms.

Medium: observe the person on a frequent basis (15min/30min).
Low: ensure whereabouts of person is known at all times.

Suicide risk (community settings, discharge, and ongoing care)

Low-risk groups of people

- Intensive follow-up (case management, telephone contacts, letters, emails, texts, home visits).
- Improved access to emergency services (crisis plan in place).

High-risk groups of people

- Intensive long-term treatment following suicide attempt.
- Short-term cognitive behavioural therapy interventions focused on problem solving.
- Interventions focused on emotional regulation, poor distress tolerance, anger management, interpersonal effectiveness, and self-esteem.

Professional objective

In any setting a professional's objective is to:

- Prevent a suicide, not just delay it.
- Focus on/enhance the thoughts of the person relating to their wish to live.
- Help the person to find alternative solutions (practical and emotional) to their difficulties and work towards recovery.
- Stop the person dying today with the hope of reducing the feeling/urge to end their life tomorrow.

Structure of detailed self-harm/suicide risk assessment

Preparing and setting the scene

- Establish a rapport.
- Use initial questions.
- Possible opening questions: 'What has brought you to the services?', 'What has been the main problem?'.

Suicidal thoughts and person's view of the future

- Check for hopelessness.
- Check for evidence of entrapment (feeling that there is no escape from the situation).
- Check for difficulty in solving problems.
- Perception of self now.
- Perception of self in future.
- Motivation for life.
- Explore suicidal thoughts, ideas, and any plans.
- Allow for revelation: allow person time to feel at ease to discuss suicidal thoughts; take what the person says seriously and acknowledge their difficulties.
- Possible exploratory questions:
  - 'Have things been getting too much for you to cope with?'
  - 'Have you ever thought that you would prefer not to face a future event?'
  - 'Have you ever thought that you would prefer not to face the next day or your current problems and difficulties?'

Clear indications of suicide

- Check for signs of suicidal intent.
- Check for preparation of suicide attempt.
- Were the plans put into place? Is there a current plan?
- Check past and current access to means.
- Was a suicide note written/left?
- Has a will recently been finalized?
- Have financial arrangements been carried out?
- Possible investigatory questions:
  - 'Have you considered any ways in which you may wish to escape from the difficulties?'
  - 'Have you made any plans about this, or preparations for it?'
- Check whether the person really wants to die.
- Was this because they wanted to escape a situation?
- Explore the persons' feelings at this time.
- Explore the persons' thoughts, are they intrusive?
- If suicidal ideation is revealed, include this in assessment and communicate immediately to others.

History of suicidal behaviour
- Ask about episodes of self-harm.
- Ask about previous attempts on their life.
- What went on?
- What were the circumstances?
- What methods were used?
- What stopped/prevented them from carrying this out?

Family history of suicide
- Check for family history of mental health/self-harm/suicidal behaviour.
- Explore any key events in family background that might be important.

Mental health difficulties
Ask and observe if the person is suffering from:
- Depression (or other common mental health problems)
- Serious mental health problems (in particular, schizophrenia)
- Alcohol problems and/or drug misuse
- Personality disorder
- Family history of suicide
- Recent contact with mental health services
- Explore: How long? How problematic?

Withdrawal and isolation
- Check for family or social network.
- Is the person living alone?
- Are they homeless?

Tests for risk of suicide
Use evidence-based accepted tests only in conjunction with full interpersonal assessment:
- Beck Depression Inventory
- Suicide Intent Scale
- Scale for Suicidal Ideation
- Beck Hopelessness Scale.

Further reading
Beck, A.T. and Weishaar, M.E. (1990). Suicide risk assessment and prediction. *Crisis* **11**(2): 22–30.

Crompton, N. and Walmsley, P. (2004). Community mental health services. In: Duffy, D. and Ryan, T. (Eds) *New Approaches to Preventing Suicide: A Manual for Practitioners*, pp. 83–98. London: Jessica Kingsley Publishers.

National Confidential Inquiry (2006). *Avoidable Deaths: five year report of the national confidential inquiry into suicide and homicide by people with mental illness*. Manchester: University of Manchester.

Pearsall, A. and Ryan, T. (2004). A&E and mental health liaison. In: Duffy, D. and Ryan, T. (Eds) *New Approaches to Preventing Suicide: A Manual for Practitioners*, pp. 54–68. London: Jessica Kingsley Publishers.

❶ Interpersonal skills

Basic personal qualities
- Self-awareness
- Empathy
- Unconditional positive regard
- Acceptance
- Communicate warmth.

Essential actions/interventions
- Establish rapport
- Active listening
- Eye contact
- Sit appropriately (position self in comfortable proximity to person)
- Consider own facial expression when responding to person.

Style of questions/intervention
- Confidentiality
- Use open questions (how, what, when, where, etc.)
- Reflect content
- Reflect feelings
- Paraphrase/check for understanding
- Feedback and sum up understanding
- Non-verbal cues.

Attitude and values
- Reflect on own attitudes towards the person and the act of self-harm.
- Consider own definition of self-harm.
- Consider own view of self-harm.
- Refrain from assuming that it is 'simply' attention seeking.
- Take what the person says seriously.
- Consider the behaviour as a possible coping strategy.
- Give time and space.
- Don't focus only on the behaviour.
- Recognize and understand nature of self-harm.

Examples of voluntary agencies in care and treatment
- Samaritans
- PAYRUS (original name: the Parents' Association for the Prevention of Young Suicide—now abbreviated to PAPYRUS Prevention of Young Suicide)
- Survivors of Bereavement by Suicide (previously known as SOBS)
- Rethink
- Campaign Against Living Miserably (CALM)
- Age Concern
- ChildLine
- Young Minds
- Depression Alliance
- Local self-harm network groups.

Final note

In most situations we can see that self-harm as an issue is not the main problem for the person—it is a behaviour or act resulting from other problems and difficulties that are causing distress for the person. From this, interventions and help should be focused on the problems that have lead to the self-harm or suicidal ideation whilst maintaining safety.

Medical emergencies

❶ Needlestick injuries

Definition
Needlestick injuries are skin punctures mainly caused by hypodermic needles, or other sharp instruments, including lancets, scalpels, or broken glass.

Physical effects
A needlestick injury allows the transmission of blood or other potentially infectious material resulting in potential exposure to blood-borne pathogens, such as the following viruses:
- Hepatitis B virus (HBV)
- Hepatitis C virus (HCV)
- Human immunodeficiency virus (HIV).

Psychological effects
The emotional impact of a needlestick injury can be traumatic and long lasting, especially during the investigation and treatment period, and even when a serious infection is not transmitted.

Safeguards
Department of Health
The standard safety procedures adopted in the UK for the prevention of needlestick injuries are known as *standard* or *universal precautions*, where all blood and body fluids—regardless of source—are considered to contain infectious agents, and are treated as such. Guidelines to this effect were published by the Department of Health in 1998.

Organizational polices
Policies and procedures are formulated at organizational level to implement the Department of Health's guidelines should be fully familiar with and abide by their employer's policies.

Prevention
Education and training about needlestick injuries is evidenced-based on research and good practice and takes place during:
- The maintenance of universal precautions which may include personal protection equipment (PPE).
- Covering one's own cuts and abrasions.
- Procedures for administrating drugs or fluids using a syringe and needle.
- The use of safer needle devices—they may cost more, but more needlestick injuries can be prevented.
- Discouraging the recapping and re-sheathing of needles.
- Undertaking risk assessments for uncooperative patients.
- Correct disposal of items into 'sharps boxes'.
- Blood-borne infection education.

Immediate actions post incident

General actions immediately after an incident:

- The wound should be encouraged to bleed freely.
- The site must be washed liberally with soap and water.
- Wounds must not be scrubbed.

Post-incident reporting

- Needlestick injuries are a major health and safety at work issue. All incidents must be recorded, monitored, and audited. The organization's policy and procedure must be followed.
- The injury should be reported *(using the organization's arrangements)* promptly to the:
  - Local manager
  - Line manager
  - Occupational Health Team
  - Infection Control Team.

Urgent advice on further management should be sought. Post-exposure prophylaxis (PEP) is generally recommended for significant exposure to blood and body fluids for HBV and HIV. PEP usually consists of:

- Hepatitis B: gammaglobulin. No prophylaxis is available for hepatitis C.
- HIV: 4 weeks of treatment with triple combination therapy using zidovudine, lamivudine, and either indinavir, nelfinavir, or soft-gel saquinavir depending on the subject's toleration of these drugs, the number of tablets associated with each regimen, interactions with any other medication, and whether the subject is pregnant.

Human bites

The most common complication of a bite is infection. Most infections are mild and can be treated with antibiotics. However, it is possible to catch tetanus which may be a potentially fatal infection. It is important to be up-to-date with your tetanus vaccinations. Human bites also carry a risk of infection from blood-borne viruses, as noted earlier.

Further reading

Expert Advisory Group on AIDS and the Advisory Group on Hepatitis (1998). *Guidance for clinical health care workers: protection against infection with blood-borne viruses.* London: Department of Health.

Health Protection Agency at ℘ http://www.hpa.org.uk/.

Needlestick Forum at ℘ http://needlestick.com/.

Royal College of Nursing (2005). *Good practice in infection prevention and control guidance for nursing staff* (Publication Code 002 74). London: RCN.

✚ Shock

Cardiogenic and hypovolaemic shock

- *Cardiogenic shock* occurs when there is not enough blood being pumped around the body. The blood supply is diverted from the surface to the core of the body. The most common cause of this type of shock is myocardial infarction (heart attack).
- *Hypovolaemic shock* occurs when the volume of blood is depleted. The most common causes are:
  - Severe blood loss, post surgery or injury.
  - Massive loss of other bodily fluids through severe diarrhoea, vomiting, or burns.
- *Septic shock* occurs as a result of severe infection and is characterized by pyrexia, rigors, and confusion.

Cardiogenic and hypovolaemic shock can both be life threatening and they are characterized by:
- Rapid pulse
- Nausea and vomiting
- Weakness and dizziness
- Rapid breathing and gasping
- Restlessness and anxiety
- Shallow respiration
- Pallor and a low blood pressure
- Skin is cold.

Treatment depends on the cause

- For blood loss, the bleeding must be stopped and a blood transfusion administered.
- For fluid loss, intravenous fluids are administered.
- Antiembolics are dangerous in some situations where there is a secondary bleeding disorder or if patients have had anticoagulation therapy.

Emergency management

- Contact medical staff.
- Do not let the person move unnecessarily, eat, drink, or smoke.
- Stay and reassure the patient.
- Treat any cause of shock which can be remedied (e.g. external bleeding).
- Lay the person down; raise and support the patient's legs.
- Remove tight clothing.
- Keep the person covered and warm if necessary.
- Record breathing, pulse, blood pressure, and level of response.
- Resuscitate person as necessary.

Anaphylactic shock (📖 Anaphylaxis)

Anaphylactic shock is an allergic reaction to:
- Food items—the main food sources for adverse reactions are nuts, peanuts, shellfish, eggs, milk, soya, wheat, and fish. Only small amounts are required to set off an adverse reaction.
- Insect bites.
- Drugs, e.g. penicillin, codeine, and aspirin.
- Other materials, e.g. latex.

Anaphylactic shock can be life threatening and the symptoms can develop very rapidly, often within a few minutes of coming into contact with the allergen. Most anaphylactic reactions occur within an hour of exposure to the causative allergen.

Characteristics
- Itching or swelling of tissues at the point where the allergen has made contact, e.g. mouth or skin around an insect bite.
- Itchiness on the scalp, palms, and/or soles of feet.
- An itchy rash that spreads over the whole body.
- The face and soft tissues can begin to swell.
- Bronchospasm.
- Oedema of the face, pharynx, and larynx.

Treatment for anaphylactic shock
Urgent action is required:
- Lay the patient flat to restore blood pressure unless they are having breathing difficulties.
- Check airways and place in recovery position.
- Check if carrying an EpiPen® or AnaPen® and help the person use it.
- Call the emergency services.

Hospital treatment may include administration of intramuscular adrenaline. This is usually stored on the 'Emergency Drug Trolley' or in a medicine cupboard in a prefilled syringe with the correct amount of adrenaline. Once adrenaline has been given recovery may be very quick.

Oxygen administration
The highest concentration oxygen should be administered immediately. The patient should be sat up in a comfortable position. Lying flat with elevated legs may be helpful for hypotension, if appropriate, but this is contraindicated if the person has breathing difficulties.

Adrenaline/epinephrine injection
- The intramuscular route is used for administering adrenaline. Monitor the patient's physical parameters as soon as possible (pulse, blood pressure, electrocardiogram (ECG), pulse oximetry).
- Patients at risk of anaphylaxis are often prescribed and given adrenaline autoinjectors (e.g. EpiPen®) for their own use.

Emotional shock
Emotional shock is a sudden or violent disturbance in the mental or emotional faculties. There are many circumstances where people may be subject to emotional shock *(witness something or be a victim of assault)* and people's resilience will vary.

Symptoms include:
- Mixed psychological reactions including fear, anxiety, anger, guilt, shame, worry, helplessness, hopelessness, numbness.
- Physical reactions, e.g. panic, tension, fatigue, fidgeting, and nausea.
- Mental state reactions, e.g. bewilderment, confusion, and disorientation.
- Panic attacks.

Emergency management

The main purpose is to assist the person to stabilize their thinking and regain a sense of control of themselves and the situation. Steps include:

- Staying with the person and providing reassurance.
- Having a plan to deal with the situation.
- Carrying out tasks for the person that they are incapable of facing at that time.

❶ Diabetes mellitus

Diabetes mellitus is a condition that occurs because of a lack of insulin in the blood or a resistance to its action, leading to a detrimental increase in blood glucose.

There are two main types of diabetes:
- Type 1 results from the body's failure to produce insulin, which requires administration of insulin.
- Type 2 results from insulin resistance, and so is non-insulin dependent and may be controlled by diet alone or with oral drugs (in some instances, however, Type 2 diabetes is treated with insulin).

Presenting features

Diabetes mellitus may present at different levels of severity:

Type 1 diabetes

Onset is usually more sudden and can affect any age group but is more common in younger people. Symptoms include:
- Constant thirst
- Increased urination
- Tiredness and weight loss
- Itchiness in the genital area
- Incidences of thrush
- Sleepiness.

Long-term complications include:
- Heart disease and strokes
- Kidney damage
- Eye retinopathy
- Foot problems.

Note: these complications may also cause medical emergencies.

Type 2 diabetes

The symptoms of type 2 diabetes mellitus may appear to be less severe and can affect any age. They include:
- Obesity
- Tiredness and lethargy
- Increased frequency of passing urine
- Itchiness/discharge in the genital area
- Increased frequency of candida albicans (thrush)

Hyperglycaemia (diabetic ketoacidosis, DKA)

DKA is potentially life threatening and occurs when the body is unable to use glucose due to the lack or absence of insulin; therefore there is an increase in fat metabolism leading to an increase in ketone bodies which cause most of the symptoms and complications (Table 4.1).

Table 4.1 Causes, signs, and management of DKA

Causes	Early signs	Emergency management
Acute illnesses and infections	Increased thirst	Carry out urine tests for ketones
Skipping or forgetting insulin or oral glucose-lowering medicine	Headaches	
	Difficulty concentrating	Continue to monitor blood glucose levels
Eating too much carbohydrate	Blurred vision	
Eating too much food and having too many calories	Frequent urination	Refer to the specialist diabetic practitioner
Infection	Fatigue (weak, tired feeling)	
Illness	Weight loss	
Increased stress	Blood glucose >180mg/dL	
Decreased activity or exercising less than usual		
Strenuous physical activity		

Hypoglycaemia

- Hypoglycaemia results from a lack of glucose in the blood (Table 4.2).
- Occurs in type 1 or type 2 (but is unusual in type 2) diabetic patients who may be familiar with early signs and symptoms which are mild enough to be managed by consuming food or drinks containing carbohydrates.

Table 4.2 Causes, signs, and management of hypoglycaemia

Causes	Early signs	Emergency management
Lack of food	Sweating	Record and monitor vital signs
Excessive exercise	Dizziness or light-headedness	Check the blood glucose level of a blood sample using a meter. If the level is less than 4 mmol/L glucose, food that includes complex carbohydrate should be consumed right away to raise blood glucose. Alternatively, the following could be administered:
Alcohol		
Overadministration of insulin	Sleepiness	
	Confusion	
	Difficulty speaking	• 3 or 4 glucose tablets • 1 sachet of glucose gel • 125mL of any fruit juice • 125mL of fizzy drink (not diet) • 250mL of milk • 1 tablespoon of sugar or honey
	Anxiety	
	Weakness	
		Recheck blood glucose in 15min to make sure it is above 4mmol/L glucose. If it's still too low, another serving of food should be eaten. These steps should be repeated until the blood glucose level is 4mmol/L glucose or above

❶ Respiratory difficulties

Breathing emergencies can result from causes such as an obstructed airway, asthma, heart failure, myocardial infarction, allergic reactions, inhaling or ingesting toxic substances, cerebrovascular accident (CVA, stroke) and, less commonly, a drug overdose reaction.

Asthma attack

Signs and symptoms

These may develop over minutes, hours, or days:
- Dyspnoea *(difficulty in breathing)* especially breathing out when wheezing can be heard
- Coughing
- Difficulty in talking
- Anxiety, distress, and panic
- Cyanosis may be present in severe cases.
- Waking at night with a persistent cough.

Emergency management

Most asthmatics are well prepared to manage attacks with the use of a prescribed reliever inhaler; however, if this is not successful within 15 minutes then the reliever must be repeated. If the patient has neb-ulised treatment prescribed, this should be administered and improve-ment monitored. Sometimes patients do not respond to treatment. If this occurs, seek urgent medical help. As a result of continuing effects of the acute episode, the person can experience extreme fatigue, dehydration, and severe hypoxia (oxygen deprivation) which in turn causes cyanosis, peripheral vascular shock, and drug intoxication from intensive therapy. Emergency medical assistance procedures need to be activated.
- Contact the doctor urgently.
- Reassurance with a calm approach is essential. Someone staying with the patient at all times will ensure this.
- Sit the patient up in a position that they find the most comfortable. Do not lie them down.
- Advise repeated use of inhaler at 5–10-min intervals via a nebuhaler, if available.
- Record breathing, pulse rate, and pulse oximetry, and repeat at 10-min intervals.
- Administer oxygen.

Hyperventilation

The person is usually unaware of overbreathing, but may feel unable to take in enough air, or that they are suffocating. They also may experience the subjective feeling of tightness in the chest, a 'lump' in the throat, and light-headedness or giddiness that in turn can cause even more appre-hension. Increased apprehension causes more overbreathing, which then increases symptoms by exacerbating chemical changes, causing more apprehension, and a vicious circle is established.

Extreme hyperventilation can result in:
- Tingling or numbness of hands, feet, and face
- Muscular twitching

- Carpopedal tetany (a syndrome characterized by flexion of ankle joints, muscular twitching, muscular cramps, and convulsions)
- Unconsciousness.

Emergency management
- Place in an upright position for comfort.
- Remove anything from the mouth, e.g. chewing gum.
- Loosen tight clothing, such as a collar, jeans, or belt.
- Offer reassurance of regaining control of breathing.
- Ask them to breathe slowly, only at about 4–6 breaths per minute.

Often, this alone will correct the problem. If this does not work, or if the person is unable to slow the breathing, re-breathing exhaled air slowly into the cupped hands, a small paper bag, or envelope may help.

If all these efforts fail, follow local emergency assistance procedures.

❶ Head injury

A head injury is trauma to the head that may or may not include injury to the brain and skull. It may be mild, moderate, or severe.

Signs and symptoms

Headache and pain at the site of the injury. If severe injury then:

- Drowsiness or loss of consciousness, slurred speech
- Double vision
- Vomiting
- Seizures
- Fluid or blood leaking from nose, ear, or mouth.

Emergency management

- Obtain some sort of history:
  - Ask witnesses
  - Has the conscious level changed since injury?
  - If the patient is initially conscious they still need observation and monitoring as it may still be a serious head injury.
  - Is there any history of fitting or airway obstruction?
  - What was the mechanism of injury and speed of any impact?
  - Be aware of any medical history and medications.
- Contact medical staff.
- Assess level of severity by undertaking neurological observations using the Glasgow Coma Scale (GCS) and continue to monitor the patient frequently. The GCS (see Table 4.3) is central to the classification, initial management, and ongoing assessment of a patient with head injuries. The maximum score is 15 and the lower the score indicates the severity of the injury:
  - Mild (GCS score 13–15)
  - Moderate (9–12)
  - Severe (<9).
- Carry out a full assessment of airway, breathing, and circulation (ABC).
- Monitor the patient closely including their temperature, pulse, respirations, blood pressure, and pupil reactions.
- Seek urgent medical help if the patient's condition deteriorates.

Table 4.3 Glasgow Coma Scale

Feature	Response	Score
Eye opening	Spontaneously	4
	To speech	3
	To pain	2
	None	1
Verbal response	Orientated	5
	Confused	4
	Inappropriate	3
	Incomprehensible	2
	None	1
Motor response	Obeys commands	6
	Localizes to pain	5
	Withdraws from pain	4
	Flexion to pain	3
	Extension to pain	2
	None	1
Maximum score		15

Record the GCS score and ensure that it is repeated regularly (every 15min). Remember that the initial neurological assessment has little value in itself. Its main use is that it provides a baseline to which subsequent scores can be compared. A decrease in the coma score of 2 or more indicates significant deterioration.

Be very careful with patients who seem to be intoxicated with alcohol (or drugs). Intoxicated people frequently sustain head injuries. Always consider that a head injury rather than intoxication might be the cause of an altered level of consciousness in this group of patients.

Glasgow Coma Scale adapted from Teasdale, G. and Jennett, B. (1974). Assessment of coma and impaired consciousness. A practical scale. *Lancet* **2**(7872):81–4. ©1974 with permission from Elsevier.

❶ Infections

Life threatening infections include:
- *Meningitis:* inflammation of the lining (meninges) of the brain and spinal cord. Bacterial meningitis is more severe than viral meningitis and can be fatal even with prompt treatment. It may attack healthy people at any age. The first symptoms can be just like flu. (Immunization can prevent bacterial meningitis.)
- *Septicaemia:* an infection of the blood, caused by bacteria or toxins entering the bloodstream, commonly known as blood poisoning. Septicaemia may present with meningitis or may present on its own.

Signs and symptoms
- General fever symptoms of pyrexia *(raised temperature)*
- Headache with or without vomiting
- Stiff neck
- Severe muscle pain
- Photophobia *(dislike of bright lights)*
- Cold hands and feet
- Stomach cramps and diarrhoea
- Very sleepy and semiconsciousness.
- Confused and irritable
- Seizures *(fits)*
- In bacterial meningitis, a rash may start as red pin pricks and develop into small bruises. An indication of septicaemia is when the rash does not disappear when a clear glass is pressed on it.

Emergency management
- Monitor and record vital signs including neurological observations.
- Seek urgent medical assistance.

Advice
Be familiar with the contents of the local infection control manual as this will advise about notifications for infectious diseases and medical emergencies procedures.

❶ Collapse and seizures

There are many reasons why a person might collapse, such as fainting, syncope, dehydration, shock, severe pain, severe infection, fever, septicaemia, hypothyroidism, postural hypotension, narcolepsy, gastrointestinal bleeding, and uncontrolled diabetes.

A thorough and comprehensive history from the patient is essential and also from witnesses. A description of the event is very helpful. Ascertain the nature, duration, and type of collapse:

- Was consciousness impaired?
- Was there a preceding aura?
- Is there a pattern to the collapse? (Exertion, time of day, after medication.)
- Are there associated symptoms? (Palpitations, headache, incontinence, seizures.)
- Has it happened before?

Stroke

A stroke is a cereberovascular accident which occurs when an area of the brain is deprived of its blood supply—usually because of a blockage or burst blood vessel. The cause may be due to cerebral ischaemia, haemorrhage, thrombosis, or embolism.

Signs and symptoms

- Facial weakness with difficulty in swallowing
- Paralysis or weakness of one side of the body
- Loss of or slurring of speech
- Sudden headache
- Blurred vision
- Loss of consciousness.

Emergency management

Follow local medical emergencies policy. Strokes are like heart attacks and require immediate medical intervention at A&E departments.

Epilepsy

Epilepsy is the paroxysmal transient disturbance of brain function that may be manifested as episodic impairment or loss of consciousness.

The seizures may be 'petit mal' *(minor)* or 'grand mal' *(severe)*. Epilepsy is controlled by medication and does not require emergency intervention unless status epilepticus occurs. This is when a seizure lasts for 30min or longer or when a person has a series of seizures and does not regain consciousness between each one.

Emergency management

- Follow hospital protocols.
- Put the patient in the recovery position if possible.
- Observe and record how the seizure affects the person.
- Monitor and record vital signs.
- Maintain airway and resuscitate if necessary.
- Maintain safety, dignity, and privacy of the patient.

Treatment

Anticonvulsant medicines and/or sedation may be administered. These must always be prescribed by the medical staff.

Further reading for all topics

Jevon, P. and Ewens, B. (2008). *Nursing medical emergency patients (essential clinical skills for nurses)*. Oxford: Blackwell Publishing Ltd.

....
....

Emergencies associated with substance misuse

❶ Problem drinking

Problems with drink can be psychological, physical, or social, and exist in varying degrees of severity. Some of the harm associated with alcohol is caused by acute intoxication and some by regular, excessive consumption over a long period. In the UK, drink problems are largely defined in terms of the harms to individuals and to society at large. Currently considerable emphasis is placed on the social harms of excessive drinking. There are in essence 3 contemporary models of problem drinking:

The Disease Model

This suggests that there is a distinction between problem drinkers and 'alcoholics' and the mass of the population who are 'normal drinkers'. The model implies that the causes of alcohol problems are to be sought in the psychological and/or physical make-up of the minority. The implication is that, short of the individual abstaining from drinking, little can be done to prevent the occurrence of the problem. Action to reduce the availability of alcohol will not be effective, only penalizing the great majority of normal drinkers who do not have problems, while failing to affect the behaviour of the small minority of problem drinkers. The best that can be done is to improve methods of identification of problem drinkers at an early stage, and ensure provision of help or treatment is available to prevent the disease progressing further.

The Integration Model

This suggests that alcohol problems arise because alcohol use is ineffectively governed by social norms, and by the existence of detrimental attitudes to alcohol use. The model suggests there is scope for primary prevention through education. It takes the view that a positive role for drink in society can be achieved by encouraging a more healthy approach to it and its place in society. It implies that if alcohol use was more effectively integrated into social and family life, so it would become an adjunct to other activities rather than an end in itself. From this standpoint, restrictions on hours of sale and age of legal consumption may be counterproductive, as they are likely to act as impediments to integrated, healthy drinking attitudes and practices.

Public Health Model ('Availability' or 'Consumption Model')

Research and experience have challenged the principal assumption and conclusions of both the Disease and Integration Models and failed to show that 'problem drinkers' share some common pre-existing psychological or physical abnormality which distinguishes them from the rest of the population. The Public Health Model is sometimes also known as the 'Availability' or 'Consumption Model' because of the key finding that the amount of alcohol-related harm in any society tends to rise and fall in line with changes in the total or average level of consumption. The more alcohol is consumed by a society, the higher its level of alcohol-related harm is likely to be. Equally, the lower its level of consumption, the lower its level of harm. This is partly because societies with a relatively high average consumption also tend to have relatively high proportions of heavy and excessive drinkers in the population.

Further reading

Edwards, G., Marshall, J., and Cook, C.C.H. (2003). *The treatment of drinking problems: a guide for the helping professions.* Cambridge: Cambridge University Press.

Heather, N. and Stockwell, T. (2004). *The essential handbook of treatment and prevention of alcohol problem.* Chichester: Wiley.

❶ Complications of alcohol misuse

The World Health Organization's Global Burden of Disease Study found that alcohol is the 3rd most important risk factor, after smoking and raised blood pressure, for European ill health and premature death. Alcohol is more important than high cholesterol levels and being overweight, 3 times more important than diabetes, and 5 times more important than asthma. In general, the higher the alcohol consumption of a country the greater the harm from alcohol. In the UK the Government advises that:

- Adult women should not regularly drink more than 2–3 units of alcohol a day.
- Adult men should not regularly drink more than 3–4 units of alcohol a day.
- Pregnant women or women trying to conceive should avoid drinking alcohol. If they do choose to drink, to protect the baby they should not drink more than 1–2 units of alcohol once or twice a week and not get drunk.

Deaths caused by alcohol consumption in the UK have doubled in the past two decades. For men who are regularly drinking more than 8 units a day (56 units/week) and women regularly drinking more than 6 units a day (42 units/week), the risks of various diseases, such as liver disease and strokes are significantly higher. For all types of alcohol-related harm, including cancers, cardiovascular diseases, and cirrhosis of the liver, the more an individual drinks, the greater the risk of harm. The annual risk of death from alcohol-related cancers (mouth, gullet, throat, and liver) increases from 14 per 100,000 for non-drinking middle-aged men to 50 per 100,000 at 4 or more units (4 glasses of wine) a day. The risk of breast cancer by age 80 years increases from 88 per 1000 non-drinking women to 133 per 1000 at 6 units a day. Risk of drinking compared with non-drinking appears to begin increasing significantly at an intake of around 3 units per day for:

- Cancers of the oral cavity and pharynx, oesophagus, larynx, breast, liver, colon, and rectum
- Liver cirrhosis
- Essential hypertension
- Chronic pancreatitis
- Injuries and violence.

Risks begin to rise with any drinking and can result in serious complications including alcoholic liver disease, the toxic effect of alcohol (acute alcohol withdrawals including seizures, delirium tremens, blackouts) or mental and behavioural disorders.

Further reading

Department of Health, Home Office, Department for Education and Skills and Department for Culture, Media and Sport (2007). *Safe. Sensible. Social. The next steps in the National Alcohol Strategy.* HMSO, London.

Prime Minister's Strategy Unit (2004). *Alcohol Harm Reduction Strategy for England.* London: HMSO.

The World Health Report (2002). *Reducing Risks, Promoting Healthy Life.* Geneva: WHO.

❶ Alcohol blackouts

Individuals experiencing blackouts often do not remember what has happened in the recent past. 'Blacking out' is not to be confused with 'passing out' or loss of consciousness. The classic cause of a blackout is heavy use of alcohol; however, surveys of drinkers experiencing blackouts have indicated that they are not directly related to the amount of alcohol consumed.

Blackouts are most likely caused by a rapid increase in a person's blood-alcohol concentration. Those with a history of blackouts are more likely to experience blackouts more frequently than others.

Occurring in association with alcohol intoxication, blackouts are periods of amnesia or forgetfulness. The phenomenon is particularly distressing especially if the person experiencing the blackout cannot remember hurting someone or behaving irresponsibly whilst intoxicated.

Often individuals have relatively intact remote memory but cannot recall events from the short term. However, other intellectual faculties often remain intact, so to the casual observer the person affected can still perform complicated tasks and seem relatively normal.

The existing literature identifies only two types of blackout: en bloc (EB) and fragmentary blackouts (FB). EBs begin and end at definitive points with full permanent amnesia for interim events, and require high blood alcohol concentrations (BACs) that disrupt limbic areas to prevent consolidation of encoded stimuli into lasting memory traces. In contrast, FBs involve a more transient, perhaps forgetful memory loss for which aspects of experience are later recalled via relatable cues.

Recent studies suggest alcohol acts at the molecular level blocking the consolidation of new memories to old memories, a process thought to include disruption of activity in the hippocampus, a brain region that plays a central role in the formation of new autobiographical memories. This characterization of alcohol-induced blackouts, however, overlooks the point that little is known about other dimensions of the construct and neglects the diversity of the nature and magnitude of the blackout experience.

Some researchers suggest blackouts are much more common among social drinkers including students and young drinkers, than previously supposed. The effects have been found to encompass events ranging from conversations to having sexual intercourse. Counselling support and education may therefore be necessary.

Further reading

Nelson, E.C., Heath, A.C., Bucholz, K.K., et al. (2004). Genetic epidemiology of alcohol-induced blackouts. *Archives of General Psychiatry* **61**(3): 257–63.

Turrisi, R., Wiersma, K.A., and Hughes, K.K. (2000). Binge-drinking-related consequences in college students: role of drinking beliefs and mother-teen communications. *Psychology of Addictive Behaviors* **14**(4): 342–55.

White, A.M. (2003). What happened? Alcohol, memory blackouts, and the brain. *Alcohol Research & Health* **27**: 186–96.

❶ Wernicke's encephalopathy

Wernicke's encephalopathy is a condition that takes its name from the 19th-century neurologist, Karl Wernicke, who first described it. Also known as 'alcoholic encephalopathy', it is an acute neurological disorder. Persistent heavy drinkers are particularly at risk, but it may also occur with thiamine (vitamin B1) deficiency states arising from other causes, particularly in patients with such gastric disorders as carcinoma, chronic gastritis, Crohn's disease, and repetitive vomiting.

The condition is characterized by a global confusional state, disinterest, inattentiveness, or agitation.

Other complications may arise including eye movement disorders (nystagmus, gaze palsies, and ophthalmoplegia, especially of the lateral rectus muscles), gait ataxia, confusion, confabulation, and short-term memory loss. Stupor and coma are rare. Gait ataxia is often a presenting symptom and in less severe cases, patients walk slowly with a broad-based gait but the gait may be so impaired as to make walking impossible.

Thiamine deficiency can also affect the temperature-regulating centre in the brainstem, which can result in hypothermia. Hypotension can be secondary to thiamine deficiency. Hypotension can also be the result of significant alcoholic liver disease.

Treatment

In its early stages it is treated with thiamine. Treatment with thiamine is often started under specialist care, although when deficiency is suspected, it should be started in primary care and followed by assessment of central nervous system and metabolic conditions.

In the 1990s there was some controversy over the safety of parentally administered thiamine with Parentrovite® preparations discontinued following a published report which warned of adverse reactions to Parentrovite®. Practice then changed to favour oral preparations. Current NHS evidence from NICE suggests there is insufficient evidence from randomized controlled clinical trials to guide clinicians in the dose, frequency, route, or duration of thiamine treatment for prophylaxis against or treatment of Wernicke's syndrome due to alcohol abuse.

Complications if untreated

Untreated, Wernicke's may progress to Korsakoff's psychosis (a brain disorder also caused by the lack of thiamine). Korsakoff's is thought to be pathophysiologically related to Wernicke's with thiamine deficiency being the pathophysiological connection. Its most common correlate is prolonged alcohol consumption resulting in thiamine deficiency. Korsakoff's is characterized by the following: retrograde amnesia (inability to recall information), anterograde amnesia (inability to assimilate new information), decreased spontaneity and initiative, and confabulation.

Further reading

Day, E. (2004). Thiamine for Wernicke–Korsakoff syndrome in people at risk from alcohol abuse. *Cochrane Database of Systematic Reviews* **1**: CD004033.

McIntosh, C., Kippen, V., Hutcheson, F., et al. (2005). Parenteral thiamine use in the prevention and treatment of Wernicke–Korsakoff syndrome. *Psychiatric Bulletin* **29**: 94–7.

❶ Acute alcohol withdrawal syndrome

The alcohol withdrawal syndrome is a cluster of symptoms observed in persons who stop drinking alcohol following continuous and heavy consumption.

Milder forms of the syndrome include tremulousness, seizures, and hallucinations, typically occurring within 6–48h after the last drink. Excessive abuse of alcohol leads to tolerance and physical reliance and a withdrawal syndrome. Unlike most withdrawals from other drugs, alcohol withdrawal can include seizures and delirium tremens and can be fatal.

Treatment

Supervised pharmacological detoxification for many years has been regarded as the standard treatment for withdrawal symptoms.

Supervised weaning from alcohol sometimes replaces medical detoxification but is not widespread practice in the UK. Heavy drinkers often struggle to come off drink without help and may require intensive medical input for a time.

To determine whether the alcohol has caused any changes or damage to the liver, it is usual to perform a liver function test (LFT). The types of proteins measured in an LFT may include some or all of the following: albumin, alkaline phosphatase (ALP), alanine transaminase (ALT), aspartate aminotransferase (AST), bilirubin and gamma-glutamyl transpeptidase (GGT).

The mean corpuscular volume (MCV) can also be used as an indicator of alcohol abuse when used alongside the results for the LFT proteins. The MCV measures the average size of the circulating red blood cells (RBCs); excessive alcohol consumption generally leads to an increase in the volume of the RBC and therefore a raised MCV measure. Further investigation is required to establish a formal diagnosis of liver disease.

Detoxification for non-complicated cases can be carried out at home or on a community-based detoxification basis.

Chlordiazepoxide is considered the 'gold standard' treatment because of its low dependence-forming potential. Daily doses of 100–200mg for a period of about 10–12 days are typical. Vitamin B compound and vitamin C may also be given.

Patients should agree a goal of longer intervention in consultation with those prescribing the detoxification regime, including whether it is suitable to pursue a goal of moderation drinking or whether it is preferable to pursue one of abstinence.

Aftercare needs to be planned for to lessen likelihood of relapse and the problem re-emerging. Detoxification with complications or with persons with complex needs should be managed with guidance from an addiction specialist. Current guidance suggests hospital admissions are only necessary if the individual has a history of delirium, seizures, temperature >38.5°C, has had a recent head injury, or is suffering from Wernicke's encephalopathy.

Further reading

DH/National Treatment Agency (2006). *Models of care for alcohol misusers (MoCAM)*. London: HMSO.
Raistrick, D., Heather, N., Godfrey, C./National Treatment Agency (NTA) (2006). *Review of the effectiveness of treatment for alcohol problems*. London: HMSO.

❶ Seizures

The relationship between alcohol and seizures is complex and multifaceted. Nonetheless, when alcohol withdrawal seizures do occur they usually do so 6–48h after sudden cessation of drinking or significant reduction in an individual's blood alcohol levels.

Seizures are more likely in those with a previous history. Metabolic disturbances due to hepatic (liver) and renal (kidney) functions may also increase the risk. Withdrawal seizures are similar to those seen with epilepsy but do not necessarily mean that someone has epilepsy.

Seizures involve a loss of consciousness of several minutes, muscle contraction and rigidity, followed by violent muscle contraction and relaxation. Other features include biting of the cheek or tongue, clenched teeth, and incontinence. In some cases breathing difficulties occur and the skin may become cyanosed (blue in colour).

Some seizures are preceded by a warning (or aura) sensation, such as characterized sounds or smells. After the seizure there may be a loss of memory, drowsiness, brief confusion, and headache. Breathing usually returns to normal soon after the end of the seizure.

Responding to seizures

First aid during a seizure involves removing sharp/hard objects from the area; protecting the head i.e. providing a cushion etc.; loosening clothing around the neck; positioning the head to prevent the tongue from obstructing the airway; and observing for difficulties.

Following the convulsion the person should be placed in the recovery position (i.e. laid on one side) to aid breathing and reduce the risk of asphyxiation. It is also important to provide reassurance and monitor the person until consciousness is regained.

It is not advisable to restrain someone during a seizure, or to put anything in the person's mouth or to force anything between his or her teeth. The person should not be moved unless they are in danger. Drinks should not be given until consciousness is fully regained.

Urgent medical attention is not always required following a withdrawal seizure, although this may be needed if an injury occurs during the seizure. Status epileptics (repeated/prolonged seizure) may cause a severe lack of oxygen to the brain and is an emergency situation requiring immediate medical attention.

To minimize the risk of a withdrawal seizure, alcohol consumption should be reduced gradually, or benzodiazepine medication, such as chlordiazepoxide or (this is the medication mentioned earlier as the gold standard treatment) diazepam should be administered.

Some long-term heavy drinkers may develop epilepsy proper and will be prone to seizures independently of alcohol withdrawal. In addition, the intoxicating effects of alcohol are increased by anti-convulsant medication, thereby increasing the risk of falls and other accidents.

Further reading

Brathen, G., Ben-Menachem, E., Brodtkorb, E., et al. (2005). EFNS guideline on the diagnosis and management of alcohol-related seizures: report of an EFNS task force. *European Journal of Neurology* **12**(8): 575–81.

Hillbom, M., Pieninkeroinen, I., and Leone, M. (2003). Seizures in alcohol-dependent patients: epidemiology, pathophysiology and management. *CNS Drugs* **17**(14): 1013–30.

❶ Delirium tremens

Delirium tremens or DTs is literally 'shaking delirium' or 'trembling madness' in Latin. DTs represent the most severe end of the spectrum of alcohol withdrawal syndromes. Concomitant sepsis, fluid and electrolyte disturbances, and recent trauma or surgery are significant risk factors for its development. DTs can be both frightening and, in severe cases, deadly

Symptoms may include uncontrollable trembling, hallucinations, severe anxiety, sweating, and sudden feelings of terror.

Treatment includes observation, comfort, care, and in some cases medication. <5% of individuals with chronic alcohol problems experience this major withdrawal symptom. It usually occurs 3–10 days after the person had their last drink.

Treatment

The goals of treatment are to save the person's life, relieve symptoms, and prevent complications. Mortality from DTs has been reduced to <5% of patients, through early diagnosis, supportive nursing care, treatment of coexisting medical conditions, and aggressive pharmacological therapy.

Patients with a history of multiple detoxification episodes are more likely to experience seizures and severe withdrawal symptoms.

Obtaining an alcohol consumption history is a critical component to identifying patients at risk and determining the appropriate treatment plan for potential alcohol withdrawal.

Nursing attention must be vigilant, with a patient preferably nursed in a separate room. IV fluid replacement may be required if there is severe sweating and dehydration. In addition, electrolyte replacement may be required.

It is essential to keep the individual calm and reduce agitation. Effective treatment is based on early recognition and sedation with benzodiazepines (diazepam or lorazepam) together with attention to concomitant illnesses. Benzodiazepines, i.e. chlordiazepoxide or diazepam, may also be used to treat alcohol withdrawal symptoms and antipsychotic medication i.e. Haloperidol may be used if the person experiences hallucinations.

Symptoms, including seizures and heart arrhythmias, may occur and will need to be treated as appropriate. The person affected may need to be put into a sedated state until withdrawal is complete.

Long-term preventive treatment may begin after the person recovers from acute symptoms. A co-worked plan of intervention between the counsellor and patient may involve a 'drying out' period, in which no alcohol is allowed.

The person should receive treatment for their alcohol problem, including counselling and advice about behaviour modifications.

The person should be tested, and if necessary, treated for other medical problems associated with alcohol use. Such problems may include alcoholic liver disease, blood clotting disorders, alcoholic neuropathy, alcoholic cardiomyopathy, and Wernicke–Korsakoff syndrome.

Further reading

Evans, K., Elder, R., and Nizette, D. (2004). *Psychiatric and mental health nursing*. New South Wales: Elsevier.

Heather, N. and Stockwell, T. (2004). The essential handbook of treatment and prevention of alcohol problem. Chichester: Wiley.

Raistrick, D., Heather, N., Godfrey, C./National Treatment Agency (NTA) (2006). *Review of the effectiveness of treatment for alcohol problems*. London: HMSO.

❶ Illegal drugs

A variety of illicit substances are taken by people, both natural and synthetic. Whilst illicit drug use often appears to be a 'modern' phenomenon, in reality psychoactive substances have been used throughout history, by nearly every human indigenous group, in religious and spiritual ceremonies, as self-medication, and for recreation. Davenport-Hines (2001) traces the history of opiate use back to early man, the first written reference found in a Sumerian text dates around 4,000 BC, predating brewing or distillation of alcohol. (Section 71 covers the classification of illegal substances, in the UK, under the Misuse of Drugs Act 1971.)

Intoxication, tolerance, and drug 'experience'

The effect a drug has on an individual is known as the *intoxicating* effect, the level that an individual becomes intoxicated is known as their *tolerance*. The degree of intoxication that a person experiences is not entirely due to the type, quantity, or strength of the drug taken. The manner in which the drug is taken (smoked, injected etc.) the individual's mood and where they are at the time of consumption as well as other intra and extra personal factors also affects their 'drug experience'. Street drugs are rarely pure and may be 'cut' with contaminants or other substances which may alter the drug experience and can pose a significant risk to the drug taker.

Categorization of drugs

A confusing array of categories exist, which drugs of abuse fall into. Dance drugs, hallucinogenics, stimulants, and opiates are common categories. Probably the most useful categories, and two which all substances fall into, are central nervous system (CNS) depressants and CNS stimulants. These are most useful because they give an indication of the properties and expected symptoms of ingestion. For example opiates (e.g. heroin, methadone, dihydrocodeine), alcohol, and benzodiazepines are CNS depressants. These effectively slow normal brain function causing shallow breathing, reducing heart rate and respiration, causing a calming effect. Crack-cocaine, amphetamines, caffeine, and khat (a herbal stimulant common in North Africa) are CNS stimulants. These increase alertness, attention, and energy, accompanied by increases in blood pressure, heart rate, and respiration.

Street names and drug 'fashion'

Colloquial names or 'street names' for drugs are common and confusingly various. Cannabis for example has been known as *blow, gear, leb, puff, marijuana, skunk, dope,* and more. (throughout the next few chapters street names are provided in italic in brackets) Some names are generic for instance in the UK, the street term, 'gear' can mean a wide variety of substances including cannabis and heroin. The names given to any substance vary locally, regionally, internationally and historically and as a result render the terms confusing and accurate identification unreliable.

Since the turn of the millennium, drug trends in the UK have shown signs of stabilization, albeit at historically high levels. Drug trends in the UK have seen types of drugs use vary and prices change. For example in the UK the price of powder cocaine has reduced, in the past two years, resulting in increasing consumption among younger people.

Preparation for use and methods of consumption

Substances of abuse can be imbibed in different ways and involve the use of a diversity of paraphernalia. In some cases substances may require preparation for consumption (e.g. heroin must be heated or 'cooked' in water with a catalyst, usually an acid, before it can be injected). The route of ingestion (e.g. smoking, eating, injecting) is important as it can render the drug more or less intoxicating.

Further reading

Davenport-Hines, R. (2001) The Pursuit of Oblivion; A Social History of Drugs. Phoenix Press, London.

Drug Scope (2007 & 2008) Street Drug Trends survey 2007 & 2008 NIDA Research report accessed at: http://www.drugabuse.gov/PDF/RRPrescription.pdf on 29/10/09

Reuter & Stevens (2007) An Analysis of UK Drug Policy; executive summary. UK drugs Policy Commission accessed at: http://www.ukdpc.org.uk/docs/UKDPC%20drug%20policy%20 review%20exec%20summary.pdf on 29/10/09

❶ Dual diagnosis

Dual diagnosis is a term first used in the USA, in the 1980s, to refer to people diagnosed with psychotic illness, who also used illicit drugs or alcohol. The term 'dual diagnosis' and co-morbidity are often used interchangeably and there is considerable debate surrounding the appropriateness of these terms to describe what is commonly a heterogeneous group of individuals with complex needs and a varied range of problems (Afuwape 2003). Today, mental health professionals have a broader understanding, and may use the term to include, someone who is depressed and drinking heavily, or using stimulant drugs (such as amphetamine or cocaine) in order to feel more socially confident. (PROGRESS 2009). The use of the term 'diagnosis' in this context is a misnomer as individuals rarely receive a formal diagnosis of both problems.

Health professionals sometimes disagree about when to apply the term. Some believe that any substance use by people with mental health problems is likely to lead to increased symptoms, and is therefore problematic. Others accept that drinking and drug use is more common amongst people with mental illness.

Prevalence: The Epidemiological Catchment Area Study, (Kessler et al. 1994; Regier et al. 1990) aimed to assess how common dual diagnosis was. 47% of the people they surveyed with schizophrenia had had a substance misuse disorder at some time in their past. The study also found the odds of having a substance misuse disorder were significantly higher amongst patients with psychotic illness than among those in the general population. In 2003 in the UK Weaver et al. found that 74.5% of drug users had a co-occuring mental health problem and 44% of psychiatric service users had a drug or alcohol problem.

Treatment: There are currently no standard treatments for dual diagnosis, largely because it ranges across such a large number of problems and can involve treatment from both substance misuse and mental health services. It's currently thought that, in the first instance, mental health services are better equipped than drug services to help people, because of their sphere of expertise. Research has demonstrated that the best prognosis is achieved through integrated treatment, where the individual receives care for their whole range of problems from a single individual or team (DH 2002).

Emergency treatment for intoxication and withdrawal from drugs or alcohol should be delivered in the same manner as for any other individual. The medium to long-term effects of both intoxication and withdrawal may include exacerbation of mental health problems and should be treated under the supervision of a psychiatric service.

Further reading

1. Afuwape, S. A. (2003) Where are we with dual diagnosis, A review of the literature. Rethink, London.
2. PROGRESS (2009) accessed at ℘ http://www.dualdiagnosis.co.uk.
3. Department of Health (2002).Mental Health Policy Implementation Guide, Dual Diagnosis Good Practice Guide.
4. Regier, D.A., Farmer, M.E., Rae, D.S., Locke, B.Z., Keith, S.J., Judd, L.L., and Goodwin, F.K. (1990) Comorbidity of mental disorders with alcohol and other drug abuse. *Journal of the American Medical Association*, 264: 2511–2518.
5. Kessler, R. C., McGonagle, K. A., Zhao, S., Nelson, C. B., Hughes, M., Eshleman, S., Wittchen, H. U., & Kendler, K. S. 1994, "Lifetime and 12-month prevalence of DSM-III-R psychiatric disorders in the United States. Results from the National Comorbidity Survey", *Arch.Gen.Psychiatry*, vol. 51, no. 1, pp. 8–19.
6. Weaver, T., Rutter, D., Madden, P., Ward, J., Stimson, G., & Renton, A. (2001) Results of a screening survey for co-morbid substance misuse amongst patients in treatment for psychotic disorders: prevalence and service needs in an inner London borough. *Social Psychiatry and Psychiatric Epidemiology* 36; 399–406.

Emergencies associated with older adults

❶ Introduction

Older adults who present to health services in an emergency usually do so due to one or more of the following factors (Fig. 6.1):
- Psychiatric
- Medical
- Social.

There is often significant overlap between these areas and it may be difficult to establish a cause–effect relationship. However, it is important to bear in mind that often what appears as a psychiatric disturbance may in fact be a medical emergency; it is therefore necessary to investigate for all possible causes before deciding on a management plan.

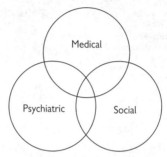

Fig. 6.1 The 3 overlapping factors for older adult emergencies.

Assessment: issues to bear in mind

Elderly patients who present via emergency services are often confused, access to their regular medical notes is lacking, and more often than not, no reliable informant is present. Therefore every effort should be made to get a good history. It is worth bearing in mind that:
- A longitudinal view is far more valuable than a cross-sectional assessment at the time of presentation.
- Additional information should be obtained from families, carers, friends, the GP, and others involved in caring for the patient in order to obtain a clear picture about the onset and progression of the illness.
- Staff who work different shifts must be consulted regarding their observations of the patient during admission, as symptoms can vary with the time of the day.
- Sleep, food, fluid, and behaviour charts, if maintained, provide important information to aid diagnosis.

❶ Psychiatric emergencies

Emergencies resulting from mental disorders include:
- Suicide and self-harm
- Self-neglect
- Harm to others and difficult behaviour.

See also 📖 Chapter 3, p. 35.

Suicide and self-harm

The spectrum of suicidal and self-harming behaviour ranges from thoughts of hopelessness, not seeing the point in being alive, wishing one were dead, ideas of harming oneself, ideas of ending one's life, planning for this, to the act of harming oneself. However, at times suicidal actions can be impulsive and unplanned, especially in psychoses.

There is often a complex interplay between biological, psychological, and social factors leading to suicidal thoughts and actions.

Suicidal thoughts in the elderly are not more common than in younger adults, but ideas of hopelessness are.

Risk factors for suicidal thoughts
- Depression
- Physical disability
- Pain
- Sensory impairment
- Institutionalization
- Being single.

Self-harm in the elderly
- To be taken seriously and treated as a suicide attempt; often the result of high suicidal intent, when compared with younger adults.
- Raises risk of further self-harm and suicide, especially in the 5 years immediately after the initial attempt.
- Overdosing is commonest method.
- Similar rates in men and women.
- Risk factors:
  - Psychiatric illness (85%)
  - Depression (>50%)
  - Alcohol misuse
  - Physical illness
  - Social isolation
  - Relationship problems
  - Bereavement
  - Male gender
  - History of previous self-harm.

Indirect self-harm

Refusal to accept treatment, food, and fluids, and avoidance of human contact may be an indirect expression of wanting to die. It may be a substitute for overt suicidal acts in the physically ill, dependent, or the cognitively impaired who cannot express their distress verbally or have no access to methods of direct self-harm. Common in:

- Very elderly
- Women
- Low-cost nursing and residential homes with high staff turnover
- Cognitive impairment
- Loss events
- Dissatisfaction with treatment
- Low religiosity.

Suicide

- Rates in UK: roughly 6 per 100,000 in those >65 years.
- Male:female ratio 3:1.
- Men adopt more violent methods (hanging—26%) than women (overdosing —36%).
- Risk factors:
  - Psychiatric illness (70%)
  - Depression (>50%)
  - Persistent feelings of hopelessness
  - Long duration of illness
  - Poor sleep
  - Alcohol misuse (<10%)
  - Schizophrenia (<10%)
  - Anxiety
  - Early dementia
  - Anxious and obsessive–compulsive personality traits
  - Male gender
  - High degree of suicidal intent
  - Previous self-harm
  - Physical illness
  - Being single
  - Limited social network
  - Relationship problems.

Assessment: issues to bear in mind

- Depressive symptoms in the elderly often present as somatic complaints.
- Physical illnesses, sensory impairment, and chronic pain, all of which are common in the elderly, are risk factors.

Self-neglect

Failure to adequately manage one's activities of daily living and achieve a reasonable level of functioning, characterized by:

- Poor food and fluid intake
- Poor personal care and hygiene
- Inadequate medication compliance
- Inadequate protection from environmental factors—inappropriate clothing, lack of heating, wandering.

Causes

Psychiatric

- Mood disorders—depression or mania
- Psychoses, e.g. schizophrenia
- Dementia
- Alcohol and other substance misuse
- Personality issues.

Medical

- Chronic pain
- Disability
- Delirium due to infective, metabolic, or endocrine causes.

Others—Diogenes syndrome

- Also known as 'senile squalor syndrome', 'social breakdown of the elderly syndrome', and 'Augean stables syndrome'.
- Not a true syndrome and no connection to the Greek philosopher Diogenes (4th-century BC).
- Often no psychiatric or medical cause.
- Commonest features:
  - Lack of personal and environmental hygiene—sometimes to the extreme extent of living amidst human or animal faeces, putrefying food, and parasitic infestations.
  - Refusal of help to remedy the situation, often coupled with denial of any problem.
  - Hoarding of usually valueless possessions and 'rubbish' (syllogomania) encroaching on living space.
- Associated features:
  - Physical illness
  - Social isolation
  - Poverty and lack of access to social care
  - Psychiatric illness
  - Personality disorders
  - Frontal lobe dysfunction.
- Prognosis: variable—some lost to follow-up, some revert to previous way of life, some go into institutional care, and may or may not accept help.

Difficult behaviour (and harm to others)

Can occur in the form of physical or verbal aggression. The behaviour may be directed and specific due to abnormal beliefs, or random and unpredictable due to hyperarousal. Seen in:

- Cognitive impairment
- Delirium
- Affective disorders—usually mania
- Psychosis.

Management of difficult behaviour

Behavioural

A detailed behavioural analysis can help find specific triggers for aggressive behaviour. Avoiding these triggers and designing the environment to reduce triggers will reduce incidents of aggression. Preferred over pharmacological interventions in dementia and delirium.

Pharmacological

Treatment of underlying psychiatric disorder.

In dementia and delirium, used only if behavioural methods of management have been unsuccessful.

The drawbacks are side effects of medication such as extrapyramidal symptoms, falls, worsening of cognition, increased risk of strokes and death with antipsychotic medication; in addition, paradoxical worsening of aggression due to disinhibition and the risk of tolerance and dependence with benzodiazepines.

- Antipsychotics:
  - Typical/1st-generation, e.g. haloperidol
  - Atypical/2nd-generation, e.g. olanzapine, risperidone, quetiapine.
- Antiepileptics—may be useful in the case of sporadic violence with no triggers:
  - Sodium valproate
  - Carbamazepine.
- Benzodiazepines—useful anti-anxiety, sedative and hypnotic agents:
  - Short acting: lorazepam
  - Long acting: diazepam.
- Cholinesterase inhibitors—some evidence of improvement in behavioural symptoms in dementia:
  - Rivastigmine—especially for psychotic symptoms in Lewy body and Parkinson's dementias
  - Donepezil
  - Galantamine
  - Memantine.
- Antidepressants and antianxiety agents may be useful if difficult behaviour is driven by depression or anxiety:
  - SSRIs such as citalopram
  - Tricyclic antidepressants, e.g. nortriptyline
  - Tetracyclic antidepressant (TCA), e.g. trazodone.

❶ Medical emergencies

As discussed previously, medical conditions may present with psychiatric symptoms and behavioural disturbance, hence it is important to be aware of these. Equally, psychiatric conditions may lead to poor self-care and poor compliance with medication, which can in turn lead to medical complications arising anew or a worsening in pre-existing medical conditions. These may occur in the community or while the elderly person is in hospital. It is necessary to treat the underlying physical cause in order to achieve remission in the behavioural and psychiatric symptoms, but these usually resolve more slowly than the physical condition.

- *Infections:* urinary infections are very common. Infections in other sites, such as the chest, wound sites, abdomen, etc. can also occur. Infections in older adults are more likely to cause a disturbance of the body's homeostasis on a background of age-compromised organ systems. This leads to symptoms of confusion, disorientation, hallucinations, and sometimes delusions.
- *Cerebrovascular:* strokes and mini-strokes (transient ischaemic attacks or TIAs) can present with confusion. Post-stroke sequelae include cognitive deficits, apathy, personality change, depression, mania, and rarely psychoses.
- *Cardiovascular:* angina and arrhythmias may present with palpitations and breathlessness which can be put down to anxiety; depression is very common after myocardial infarction (MI) and is a poor prognostic factor for recovery after an MI. Arrhythmias can lead to poor brain perfusion and to cognitive deficits.
- *Metabolic:* disturbances in electrolyte or glucose levels can present as delirium, altered behaviour, or psychosis.
- *Neoplasms:* tumours of the central nervous system can directly affect the brain due to pressure or inflammation of surrounding tissues and result in cognitive dysfunction, depression, or psychotic symptoms. Tumours elsewhere in the body can also cause these symptoms via inflammatory or metabolic disturbances or by releasing substances which cause paraneoplastic syndromes.
- *Iatrogenic:* therapeutic procedures or agents may cause confusion (e.g. postoperative) or mood or psychotic symptoms (e.g. steroid-induced psychosis, depression, or mania).
- *Falls:* any of the conditions in this list may result in falls; psychiatric conditions leading to worsening of physical health and psychotropic or other drugs may lead to falls. Falls leading to head injury or wounds and infections may subsequently lead to confusional states.
- *Constipation:* not usually a medical emergency, constipation can, however, be a potent and easily overlooked cause of confusion. Immobile or cognitively impaired patients are particularly at risk.

❶ Social emergencies

These can result directly from social, medical, or psychiatric causes or indirectly as a result of increased vulnerability from them.

- Homelessness or unsuitable living conditions secondary to:
  - Self-neglect
  - Psychiatric disorder
  - Cognitive decline
  - Poverty
  - Social isolation.
- Relationship breakdowns due to:
  - Psychiatric disorders—mania and psychoses
  - Changes in personality and difficult behaviour in dementia
  - Loss of a spouse or partner who acted as a social link.
- Bereavement:
  - Can result in social isolation, precipitate the onset of psychiatric illness, and lead to worsening physical health and self-neglect.
- Elder abuse: single or multiple acts or lack of action occurring in a relationship where there is an expectation of trust, leading to harm to the elderly person. Look for the following signs:
  - Physical: unexplained injuries, clusters of injuries, injuries at different stages of healing, medication misuse (e.g. excessive use of sedatives).
  - Sexual: perineal lesions, bleeding from rectum or vagina, difficulties in walking, sitting.
  - Emotional: anxiety, agitation, passivity, apathy, or unexplained origin.
  - Financial: inexplicable transactions, e.g. large withdrawals that do not match lifestyle, sudden inability to pay bills, etc.
- Financial vulnerability due to poor judgement, altered mental state (e.g. mania) or poor cognition (e.g. dementia):
  - Debts
  - Poor financial judgement and excessive expenditure
  - Exploitation by others—see earlier in list.

Management of social emergencies requires cooperation between the disciplines of medicine, psychiatry, and social services. After assessment for any medical and psychiatric disorders—and treatment of these if appropriate—social services would need to provide their input to find safe and appropriate accommodation for these patients.

ⓘ Delirium

Also known as acute confusional state. Characterized by:
- Altered consciousness (qualitative and quantitative):
  - Reduced awareness of environment
  - Reduced ability to focus, sustain, or shift attention.
- Impaired recall and immediate memory with relatively preserved longer-term memory.
- Disorientation to time, place, and person.
- Psychomotor disturbances:
  - Reduced or increased activity and speech
  - Enhanced startle response
  - Increased reaction time.
- Circadian rhythm disturbances:
  - Insomnia
  - Daytime drowsiness
  - Reversal of sleep–wake cycle
  - Nocturnal worsening of symptoms.
- Rapid onset and fluctuating course.
- Evidence that there is underlying physical cause.
- Emotional lability and behavioural changes.

Epidemiology
- 30% inpatients >65 years
- 1–2% of community patients >65 years
- 14% of community patients >85 years
- 2/3 unrecognized.

Causes
- Infection: 33%
- Metabolic disturbance (e.g. 10% after MI, postoperative, post-stroke)
- Endocrine abnormality (e.g. diabetes, Cushing's)
- Toxic: DTs—10%
- Post-traumatic
- Multiple causes: 25%.

Risk factors
- Increasing age
- Dementia
- Previous episode of delirium
- Being on >3 drugs
- Psychoactive substances
- Dehydration
- Sensory impairment
- Bladder catheter.

Management

- Promptly investigate for and treat underlying cause.
- General supportive measures such as rehydration, preventing malnutrition, preventing pressure sores.
- Treat constipation if present.
- Promote orientation through clocks, calendars, name boards; avoid frequent changes of wards, beds, and staff.
- Promote sleep, eliminate noise, and minimize sensory impairment with hearing aids, spectacles, etc.
- In hypoactive delirium, reduce sedating medication.
- In hyperactive delirium, benzodiazepines and antipsychotics in low doses and cholinesterase inhibitors may be used to manage behavioural disturbance.

❶ Degenerative disorders: dementias

Characterized by
- Decline in memory, usually of recent memory and later of longer-term memories.
- Decline in other cognitive abilities such as judgement, planning, organization, language, visuospatial skills, perceptual skills.
- Preserved awareness of environment (no clouding of consciousness, unlike in delirium).
- Delusions and hallucinations.
- Altered behaviour/change in personality in the form of:
  - Emotional lability
  - Agitation
  - Irritability and aggression
  - Coarsening of social behaviour.

The last two are often referred to as behavioural and psychiatric symptoms of dementia (BPSD).

Epidemiology

Prevalence increases exponentially with age:
- Rare under the age of 60
- 1% at 60–64 years
- 1.5% at 65–69 years
- 3% at 70–74 years
- 6% at 75–79 years
- 13% at 80–84 years
- 24% at 85–89 years
- 34% at 90–94 years
- 45% at >95 years.

Risk factors

- Increasing age – by far the most important (see 'Epidemiology', p. 92)
- Female gender
- Genetic factors
- Smoking
- Alcohol intake
- Obesity
- Hypertension
- Dyslipidaemia
- Stroke
- Heart disease
- Low education
- Low socioeconomic status
- Depression
- Head injury
- Chronic inflammation
- Vitamin deficiency.

Protective factors

- Mentally stimulating activity
- Physical activity
- Good social networks
- Leisure activity
- Antihypertensive therapy
- Anti-inflammatory treatment
- Hormone-replacement therapy
- Adequate nutrition.

Types of dementia

Alzheimer's (60%)

- Most common cause of dementia.
- Increasing incidence with age; rare forms of early onset dementia due to genetic causes.
- Characterized by brain atrophy and pathological brain changes neurofibrillary tangles and senile plaques which are the result of accumulation of abnormal proteins.
- Usually insidious onset and gradual progression.
- Typically starts with episodic memory impairment and progresses to global cognitive dysfunction.
- Neurological signs are uncommon early in the illness.

Vascular (15–20%)

- Caused by ischaemic and haemorrhagic brain lesions due to hypoxic brain damage (multi-infarct dementia) or prolonged hypoperfusion of brain areas leading to changes in white matter (small-vessel disease).
- History is often of abrupt onset and 'step-wise' deterioration, corresponding to vascular events.
- Deficits in speech, visuospatial, and perceptual difficulties may be present before memory loss.
- Neurological signs are often present.
- Often found together with evidence of Alzheimer's disease—so-called mixed dementia.

Lewy body/Parkinson's disease dementia (LBD)

- Caused by accumulation of Lewy bodies inside neuronal cells.
- Similar pathology is found in Parkinson's disease, which can later progress to dementia; LBD and Parkinson's are thought to be on the same spectrum of illnesses, with more prominent psychiatric and neurological symptoms respectively.
- Characterized by fluctuating cognitive deficits, recurrent visual hallucinations, REM sleep behaviour disorder, parkinsonian features, and severe sensitivity to antipsychotic medication.
- Memory impairment may be less than visuospatial and frontal deficits

Fronto-temporal dementia (FTD)

- Atrophy of frontal and temporal brain areas.
- Age of onset usually <65 years.

- Onset is insidious, with subtle changes in language and personality being early symptoms; rigidity of behaviour, overeating and preference for sweet food seen.
- Episodic memory, visuospatial and visuoperceptual skills are usually preserved, with significant deficits in language and frontal lobe function.

Less common causes of dementia
- Alcohol related (history of significant alcohol use and demonstrable link to dementia).
- Huntington's disease (autosomal dominant hereditary neurological disease characterized by movement disorders, dementia and psychiatric symptoms).
- Multiple sclerosis.
- Creutzfeldt–Jakob disease: CJD—a prion disease with age of onset around 65 years, catastrophic progression, and additional neurological signs such as myoclonus and characteristic electroencephalogram (EEG) changes; death occurs within 1 year.
  - A variant form, vCJD, affects younger adults aged 20–40, presents with peripheral neurological signs and cognitive decline, EEG may be normal in early stages; decline is rapid, death within 2 years)
- HIV dementia: a late manifestation of AIDS with global cognitive impairment and multiple psychiatric symptoms, often in severely immunosuppressed patients.

Diagnosis
- Detailed clinical history, with collateral history.
- Cognitive testing using the Mini Mental State Examination (MMSE) or Addenbrooke's Cognitive Examination – Revised (ACE-R) or other standardized test.
- Physical, especially neurological examination.

Investigations
- Blood tests: FBC, U&Es, LFTs, renal function, TFTs, bone profile, iron studies, glucose, lipid profile, vitamin B12, and folate levels.
- Computed tomography (CT) or magnetic resonance imaging (MRI) head scan will reveal areas of atrophy, vascular changes and rule out other lesions such as tumours.

Management
Non-pharmacological
- Support, adaptation, and adjustment of living environment and care needs taking into account the decline in cognitive abilities and functioning.
- Minimizing risks identified, e.g. by occupational therapy.
- Psychoeducation—planning for the future, e.g. power of attorney, advance decisions, etc.
- Carer support—education, social care, respite.
- Management of difficult behaviour (see 📖 Difficult behaviour (and harm to others, p. 87)).

Pharmacological—to slow the rate of cognitive decline and for management of BPSD
- Cholinesterase inhibitors: donepezil, galantamine, and rivastigmine—the last being licensed for treatment of visual hallucinations in LBD.
- NMDA receptor antagonist: memantine.

Treatment of coexisting conditions
- Antidepressants for depression.
- Antianxiety agents.
- Antipsychotics—with caution as increased risk of stroke and death; caution in LBD.
- Vascular protection—antihypertensives, statins for dyslipidaemias, antiarrhythmics.

❶ Depression

Core symptoms: (2 of 3 must be present in mild and moderate depression and all 3 in severe depression):
- Low mood
- Loss of interest or pleasure in activities normally pleasurable (anhedonia)
- Low energy or increased fatigability.

Additional symptoms: (2, 4, or 5 symptoms must be present in mild, moderate, or severe depression respectively):
- Loss of self-confidence
- Excessive and inappropriate guilt or self-reproach
- Recurrent thoughts of death or suicide, or suicidal behaviour
- Decreased concentration or ability to think—indecisiveness, vacillation
- Psychomotor retardation or agitation
- Sleep disturbance
- Appetite change.

Epidemiology

1–4% of community dwellers >65 years meet criteria for 'major depression', but 9–14% have clinically significant depressive symptoms not meeting strict diagnostic criteria.

Risk factors
- Physical illness
- Residence in nursing homes (3 times higher)
- Hospitalization
- Cognitive impairment
- Genetic factors
- Female gender
- Being single
- Past psychiatric history
- Personality issues.

Assessment: in comparison with younger adults
- Somatic complaints more common
- Hypochondriasis more likely
- More psychomotor disturbance
- Greater likelihood of psychotic symptoms
- Less irritability and hypersomnia
- More insomnia.

Management
Physical
- Pharmacological: antidepressant drugs such as selective serotonin reuptake inhibitors (SSRIs), TCAs.
- Electroconvulsive therapy (ECT), especially for severe, psychotic depression; most rapid clinical response.

Psychological
Cognitive behavioural therapy, interpersonal therapy, psychodynamic psychotherapy, etc.

❶ Mania

Symptoms
- Increased physical activity
- Increased talkativeness
- Racing thoughts
- Difficulty in concentration and increased distractibility
- Decreased need for sleep
- Increased sexual energy and promiscuity
- Spending sprees, other reckless or socially inappropriate behaviour
- Inflated self-esteem and grandiosity
- In a milder form—hypomania
- In a more severe form with delusions and hallucinations—mania with psychotic features.
- No specific differences from mania in younger adults, but can sometimes be difficult to distinguish from delirium.
- Age of onset >50 years—late-onset mania.

Neurological comorbidity associated with manic syndromes in late onset mania:
- Right-brain lesions
- Cerebrovascular disease
- Head injuries
- Endocrine disorders
- HIV
- Epilepsy.

Management
- Investigate for and treat comorbid medical conditions in late onset mania.
- Mood stabilizers: lithium, valproic acid, carbamazepine, gabapentin, lamotrigine.
- Antipsychotics: to treat acute phases of mania—beware side effects and risks discussed previously.

❶ Psychoses

Late-onset schizophrenia (onset >40 years), very late-onset schizophrenia-like psychosis (onset >60 years), and paraphrenia are terms used to describe psychotic disorders in older adults, based on age of onset, presence or absence of cognitive deficits, and similarity of symptoms to classic schizophrenia. However, the symptoms these illnesses have in common are:

- Delusions—firmly held false beliefs. These can be of the following types:
  - Self-reference: 76%
  - Control (by an external agency): 25%
  - Grandiose ability: 12%
  - Hypochondriacal nature: 11%
  - Persecution
- Hallucinations: auditory, visual, olfactory, gustatory, or somatic
- Mood symptoms: depression in up to 60%, more in women
- Cognitive deficits.

Risk factors
- Positive family history
- Female gender
- Structural brain abnormality: strokes etc.
- Sensory deficits: deafness (40% of late paraphrenia), visual impairment
- Abnormal personality: schizoid or paranoid types.

Management
- Pharmacological—antipsychotics:
  - 2nd-generation or atypical—olanzapine, risperidone, quetiapine, clozapine.
  - 1st-generation or typical—haloperidol, trifluoperazine, chlorpromazine.
- Psychosocial—building a therapeutic relationship, re-housing etc.

❶ Substance misuse

Substance misuse disorders in the elderly are commonly under-recognized and underestimated as the focus of research, treatment, and public health initiatives in this field is towards younger adults.

They are characterized by 1 or more of the following:

- Acute intoxication (excessive use of a substance, signs and symptoms consistent with excessive use, which cannot be explained by another disorder).
- Harmful use (substance is responsible for or contributes to substantial physical or mental harm, the pattern of use persists for >1 month or occurs repeatedly over 12 months).
- Dependence syndrome (strong desire to use the substance, impaired ability to control use, withdrawal reaction—see later, tolerance to the effects of the substance and needing higher doses to achieve the same effect, preoccupation with substance use, and persisting in the use despite harmful consequences).
- Withdrawal syndrome (cessation of use in prolonged and/high doses leads to signs and symptoms that result from withdrawal from the particular substance, and these are not explained by the presence of any other medical disorder) e.g. DTs in alcohol withdrawal.

Acute intoxication and withdrawal states may present as medical and psychiatric emergencies, e.g. DTs present with hallucinations, delusions, fluctuating cognition, fever, tachycardia, autonomic instability (rapidly varying pulse and blood pressure) and dehydration. The treatment is in a medical setting, with IV fluids, IV thiamine, and multivitamins, general nursing and benzodiazepine detoxification.

Older adults commonly misuse alcohol and medication (prescribed or over the counter); illicit drug use is not usual. However, generations of people reaching the age of 65 are likely to continue drug-use patterns over the next few decades.

Risk factors

- Family history
- Previous substance use
- Personality traits
- Gender (men: alcohol and illicit substances; women: sedative hypnotics and anxiolytics)
- Chronic illness and pain: opioid analgesics
- Long-term prescribing without review: sedative hypnotics, anxiolytics
- Care-giver over use of as needed medication
- Stress, loss, social isolation
- Psychiatric disorders.

Assessment and management

- Look for evidence of dependence, other psychiatric condition, e.g. depression, evidence of social harm (e.g. debt, relationships, legal problems).
- Physical examination and investigations, especially vitamin B12, folate and liver function.
- Detox if required.
- Vitamin bolus and supplements.
- Advice and education about alcohol and drugs.
- Work towards abstinence and prevention of relapses.
- Consider referral to specialist alcohol service.

❶ Legal issues

Legislation varies across the UK, what follows is a brief description of the laws in England that might applicable in emergency situations. (See also 📖 Chapter 9, p. 161.)

Mental Health Act (MHA) 1983 (amended 2007)—England

- Provides for detention (for assessment or treatment of) or supervised community treatment of persons with a mental disorder.
- No age limit.
- To minimize undesirable effects of mental disorder, maximize safety and well-being of patients, promote their recovery, and prevent harm to others.
- Guiding principles are least restrictive option, patient participation, protection of patient rights and respect for diversity of lifestyles.

Mental Capacity Act (MCA) 2005—England and Wales

- Provides a legal framework for making decisions on behalf of individuals who lack the mental capacity to make those decisions for themselves.
- Applicable to persons aged 16 and over (age of presumption of capacity).

Statutory principles

- Presumption of capacity unless proved otherwise.
- All possible steps must be taken to enhance capacity.
- Capacity must not be questioned only because the decision seems unwise.
- Decisions must be in the best interest of the person.
- Objectives cannot be achieved by less restrictive options.

Capacity assessments

- Are decision- and time-specific.
- Lack of capacity—a person must be unable to:
  - Understand and believe the information relevant to the decision.
  - To retain the information (even if for a short period of time).
  - To use or weigh up the information in the decision-making process.
  - To communicate the decision.

MCA also covers advance directives to refuse treatment in case of future loss of capacity—decisions to refuse life-sustaining treatments must be made in writing.

Deprivation of Liberty Safeguards (DoLS) 2008

- To provide a legal framework around the deprivation of liberty, and prevent breaches of the European Commission on Human Rights (ECHR).
- Doesn't apply to those under MHA.
- Must be for person's protection, in their best interests, proportionate to the likelihood of harm, least restrictive option, for the least possible time, must be authorized be a 'supervising body'.
- E.g. person with dementia in a care home.

Lasting Power of Attorney (LPA)—England and Wales

- An 'attorney' can be appointed to act for them by persons (donors) who fear loss of capacity in the future.
- Can be for property and affairs (individuals or firms) or personal welfare (individuals only).
- Must be registered with the Office of the Public Guardian.
- Attorneys must always act in the best interest of the donors.

Do Not Resuscitate (DNR) decisions

- Made when:
  - CPR will not restart the heart or breathing.
  - Treatment is of no benefit to the patient as it will result in poor quality of life.
  - Benefits are outweighed by burdens.
  - A person has previously consistently stated their wish not to be resuscitated.
  - A person has made an advanced directive against life-sustaining treatment.
- Must be made in discussion with patients, their families or carers.
- Must be made by a senior clinician.

Further reading

Jacoby, R., Oppenheimer, C., Dening, T., et al. (Eds.) (2008). Oxford Textbook of Old Age Psychiatry. Oxford: Oxford University Press.

Department of Constitutional Affairs. (2007). Mental Capacity Act 2005: Code of Practice. London: TSO. Available at: ℘ http://www.dca.gov.uk/legal-policy/mental-capacity/mca-cp.pdf

Department of Health (2008). Code of Practice: Mental Health Act 1983. London: TSO. Available at: ℘ http://www.dh.gov.uk/prod_consum_dh/groups/dh_digitalassets/@dh/@en/documents/digitalasset/dh_087073.pdf

National Institute for Health and Clinical Excellence. (2006). Dementia: supporting people with dementia and their carers in health and social care. London: NICE. Available at: ℘ http://www.nice.org.uk/nicemedia/live/10998/30318/30318.pdf

Emergencies associated with children

❶ Crisis: responses

Crisis theory

A crisis can occur to anyone and usually indicates that a person's normal coping strategies cannot deal with the situation they are faced with. Geral Caplan developed the theory of crisis in his study of grief reaction and bereavement. All crises have some elements of a common theme such as:

- Initial reaction shock and an increase in anxiety.
- Individual tries to use normal coping strategies and if they don't work the crisis will continue.
- Asking for help.
- Some kind of adaptation is achieved which can benefit the individual or not.

Types of crisis

Crises fall into 3 broad categories:
- Development crises
- Situational crises
- Traumatic crises.

Methology

Brammer illustrates a 4-step problem-solving approach to crisis intervention:

- A comprehensive assessment of factors contributing to the crisis, assessment of risk, the individual view of the crisis, assessment of coping skills and social networks to contain the crisis.
- Planning involves nurse and client working together to define the problem, examining existing coping skills, introducing new coping skills, involvement of social networks, and emphasizing that the problem can be overcome.
- Implementation involves the nurse demonstrating a willingness to help and includes interventions which directly help the individual resolve the problem or directly change the individual's environment by removing them from the situation.
- Evaluation should be done jointly by those involved and should look at the successful and unsuccessful outcomes.

Fundamentals of crisis intervention

- Communication is key to crisis intervention and includes flexibility in preference to the environment a client wishes to be seen, listening to what the client is saying, showing respect and making the client feel valued, above all, communicating allows the individual to form a therapeutic relationship which is the vehicle for change.
- Flexibility also involves the acceptance that crises do not happen between 9–5 and that clients involved in crises are often chaotic. This involves not only a flexible approach to working hours and location but also a holistic approach of nursing to meet client needs.
- Working within a team also provides for crisis intervention by allowing for a collaborative approach to crisis management and reflective practice.

Further reading

Brammer, L.M. (1979). *The helping relationship: Process and skills*. Englewood Cliffs, NJ: Prentice Hall.

Caplan, G. (1964). *An Approach to Community Mental Health*. New York: Grune & Stratton.

❶ Diagnostics and labelling

Diagnostics

Diagnosis

Diagnosis refers to the process of identifying a medical condition or disease by its signs, symptoms, and from various diagnostic procedures. The majority of mental health professionals refer to the ICD-10 (International Classification of Diseases) when making diagnoses of psychiatric disorder. However, many feel that adult diagnostic criteria are inappropriate for children as developmental issues influence the symptoms of psychiatric disorders and it is vital that those making diagnoses have the special knowledge and skills in working with children and young people.

The diagnostic process is more than attributing a label and a classification code, treatment effectiveness depends on the quality of the clinician–patient relationship as well as on the nature of the disorder. Clinicians must approach the child/young person with genuine honesty and interest. If a child/young person is meaningfully engaged in a relationship, the diagnostic process not only provides clinical understanding but establishes an alliance pivotal to treatment success.

Emergency situations

In an emergency situation, when faced with a patient for the very first time, the most important factors to consider are engagement and risk assessment. Risk assessment is essentially a diagnostic assessment technique which gleans information from various sources about the current situation and presentation.

Risk assessment is the beginning of the identification of symptoms which aids the diagnostic process, which in turn leads to the formulation of management and treatment plans. A psychiatric diagnosis is necessary but not sufficient information on which to base a treatment plan; the diagnosis can tell us only a small part of what we need to know. By completing a comprehensive risk assessment not only will the diagnostic process have begun but clear and comprehensive management and treatment plans can be implemented.

Labelling

Unfortunately, mental illness often attracts fear, hostility, and disapproval rather than compassion, support, and understanding. Once identified as different it can be hard for an individual to be accepted, and in childhood and adolescence this can have profound effects, especially when relationships with peers are of huge importance.

It is essential that mental health professionals within their roles not only support children and young people in accepting and living with their diagnoses but also educate the wider public on mental health issues in order to destigmatize the negative attitudes and beliefs held around mental health.

❶ Sexual exposure

The most likely situations the clinician will face are:
- 1. Disclosures by children that they have been sexually abused (remember that 'sexual abuse' does not necessarily involve contact and includes, for instance, being shown pornography by an adult or witnessing adult sex).
- 2. Receiving information that a child has done something sexually harmful to another child (or adult).
- 3. Hearing that a young person has consented to a sexual experience with another.
- 4. Being informed that a child has obtained pornographic images, or is engaged in sexualized communication via the Internet or mobile phone.

In all of these categories there is a possibility that a criminal offence has been committed and/or a safeguarding issue is at stake. Wherever this is possible then the clinician must:
- Discuss the information obtained with a more senior colleague, and
- Consult the local safeguarding (child protection) procedures which will define the action to be taken and could well involve contacting the police or Children's Services.

In addition, your own agency will probably have a child protection specialist who is available for consultation and who will need to be informed. Looking at each of the above categories in turn:
- 1. It is unusual for a child to make a disclosure of sexual abuse out of the blue. A more common situation is that there are growing suspicions because of a child's behaviour, such as:
  - Involvement in high-risk sexual behaviour, or the opposite, sexual avoidance.
  - Absconding from home or risk-taking behaviour.
  - Harming others, physically or sexually.
  - Self-harm.

The child will need a high level of trust in the clinician before information about sexual abuse is passed on. To avoid 'contamination of evidence', it is advisable to obtain sufficient information only to satisfy yourself that abuse has occurred, before handing over to police/Social Services.
- 2. Two important findings from research to emerge in recent years are:
  - Young children, e.g. 4-year-olds, who engage in sexually concerning behaviour are very likely to have been sexually abused themselves, but the older the child, the less likely this is so.
  - Young people who sexually harm or offend are unlikely to repeat their behaviour. One study found recidivism rates of between 5–18%.
- 3. The issue of whether the sexual contact was by consent needs to be explored in detail:
  - Was there a power imbalance between the pair?
  - Was there coercion, however subtle?
  - Use of bribes?

Any sexual contact where one of the parties is under 16 years is technically a criminal offence.

- 4. Modern modes of communication have exposed children and young people to greater potential for viewing pornography and sexualized messaging. In assessing whether further action should be taken consider:
  - The nature of the indecent material (the Sentencing Advisory Panel, 2002, devised a 5-point scale ranging from, level 1—erotic posing with no sexual activity, to level 5—sadism or bestiality).
  - The extent of the individual's involvement with it.
  - Whether another party has been injured by the activity (e.g. transmitting an indecent image of a person without their consent).
  - Whether the child could be the victim of an internet predator.

Current legislation covering sex offences is provided by the Sexual Offences Act 2003. More detail can be found online.

Further reading

Burton, D.L. (2000). Were adolescent sexual offenders children with sexual behaviour problems? *Sexual Abuse* **12**(1): 37–48.

Worling, J. and Curwen. T. (2000). Adolescent sex offender recidivism: success of specialised treatment and implications for risk prediction. *Child Abuse and Neglect* **24**: 965–82.

❶ Drugs and alcohol

Overview

Substance misuse in young people is similar to that of adults in that they take substances for their stimulant, sedative, or hallucinogenic effects. However, on the whole, adolescent drug taking is significantly dissimilar.

Aetiological factors, patterns of use, context of use, personal, and developmental differences make it necessary to take different pharmacological and psychosocial treatment approaches. Adult substance misusers often present to services at the later stages of the addiction process, usually when experiencing physical and/or psychological dependence. Adolescents are usually at an earlier stage of this process, therefore detoxification is rarely needed and rehabilitation often is.

For most adolescents, drug and/or alcohol taking tends to be the most visible symptom of a range of other difficulties. Adolescents who have drug/alcohol misuse of sufficient severity to require treatment are likely to be struggling with the developmental tasks of adolescence and their drug taking is usually part of a network of interconnected issues and problems which can impair their transition into adult life. Intoxication can act as a disinhibiting influence that can increase the likelihood of aggressive behaviour and/or antisocial behaviour. Funding of substances is often through criminal activity, both non-violent crimes such as shoplifting and violent crime such as street robbery. Young people tend to use substances out of curiosity with multiple substances being used more frequently rather than the exception. They are more likely to exhibit binges and are usually affected by consequences of acute intoxication rather than chronic use.

Challenges

- Ethical, legal, and child protection safeguarding issues.
- Engagement and retention into services.
- Chaotic lifestyle as a result of living with dependent drug users and/or exposure to criminal activity, e.g. drug dealing.
- Developmental issues which can impede on facilitating disclosure.
- Self-medicating, e.g. attention deficit hyperactivity disorder (ADHD).
- Diagnostic issues overlap between mental health, substance misuse, and behaviour.
- High risk of accidental overdose and/or suicide due to inconsistent, exaggerated, or minimizing responses about the amount, frequency, and unknown substances being used. Often reluctance to give urine sample to confirm substance use.
- Injecting drug use increases the risks of accidental overdose as well as volatile substance use, such as petrol and gas being linked to high levels of accidental death.
- Review and monitoring of prescribed medication to minimize the risk of accidental overdose.
- Behavioural risks associated with stimulants and alcohol misuse may lead to disinhibition, increasing potential for aggression, self-harm, and unprotected sex increasing the risk of teenage pregnancy.

- Exposure to blood-borne viruses, physical health problems, withdrawal symptoms.
- Changing cultural and economic factors, e.g. gang culture, increased availability/decreased price of alcohol, and relative reduction in the street price of drugs.
- Increasingly more potent drugs available, e.g. skunk, methamphetamine.
- Language of drug taking, e.g. 'bag', 'points', 'teenths'.
- Limited evidence-based practice and training issues.

Further reading

Crome, I.B. (1999). Treatment interventions looking towards the millennium. *Drug and Alcohol Dependence* **55**: 247–63.

Crome, I., Ghodse, H., Gilvarry, E., *et al.* (2004). *Young People and Substance Misuse*. London: Royal College of Psychiatrists.

Ungerleider, J.T. and Segel, N.J. (1990). The drug abusing adolescent: clinical issues. *Psychiatric Clinics of North America* **13**: 435–42.

❶ Asperger's syndrome

Asperger's syndrome (also called Asperger's disorder, Asperger's, or AS) is an autism spectrum disorder (ASD). It is a developmental disorder that is due to abnormalities in the way the brain develops and functions.

It is characterized by difficulties in social interaction and restricted, stereotyped patterns of behaviour and interests.

People with AS can find it harder to read the signals that most of us take for granted. This means they find it more difficult to communicate and interact with others which can lead to high levels of anxiety and confusion

Pursuit of specific and narrow areas of interest is one of the most striking features of AS

Diagnosis

- Most parents find that obtaining a correct diagnosis is an important first step.
- Diagnosis is most commonly made between the ages of 4–11 years.
- Delayed or mistaken diagnosis can be traumatic for individuals and families.

Challenges

- Children with AS often display behaviour, interests, and activities that are restricted and repetitive and are sometimes abnormally intense or focused.
- Problems can arise when these obsessions can be socially unacceptable or even break the law. However, the hypothesis that individuals with AS are predisposed to violent or criminal behaviour has been investigated but is not supported by data.
- Children with AS prefer familiar routine and tend to resist change, which they find difficult and unpleasant.
- AS treatment attempts to manage distressing symptoms and to teach age-appropriate social, communication, and vocational skills that are not naturally acquired during development, with intervention tailored to the needs of the individual child.
- Children with AS have an increased prevalence of comorbid psychiatric conditions such as ADHD, depression, and anxiety and treating these can be a challenge.
- Medication can be effective in combination with behavioural interventions and environmental accommodations in treating comorbid symptoms; however, no medications directly treat the core symptoms of AS.
- Stress and anxiety can present as inattention, withdrawal, reliance on obsessions, hyperactivity, or aggressive or oppositional behaviour.
- Adolescents with AS may exhibit ongoing difficulty with self-care, organization, and disturbances in social and romantic relationships.
- Most individuals with AS can learn to cope with their differences, but may continue to need moral support and encouragement to maintain an independent life.

Further reading

McPartland, J. and Klin, A. (2006). Asperger's syndrome. *Adolescent Medicine Clinics* **17**(3): 771–88.

Rutter, M. and Taylor, E. (Eds.) (2002). *Child and Adolescent Psychiatry* (4th edn). London: Blackwell.

❶ Autism

Autism is a developmental disorder that shows itself in the first 3 years of life and is due to abnormalities in the way the brain develops and functions.

Challenges

Socializing

Children with autism tend to ignore other people or appear insensitive to others' needs, thoughts, or feelings. They do not make the usual eye contact or use facial expression in social situations. They tend to find it difficult to cooperate, share, or take turns with others. They prefer to play alone, and show no interest in imaginative play. Socializing with other children and forming friendships is hard for them.

Communication difficulties

Not being able to communicate properly is a particularly disabling aspect of autism, and often the one that first causes concern. Nearly all affected children have language problems—both in understanding and in speaking. More severely affected children might never learn to speak or to communicate in other ways.

Difficulties with expressive communication may lead autistic children to become frustrated. This frustration may lead to expression through excited behaviour, screaming, crying, tantrums, acts of aggression, and/or self-abuse.

Unusual behaviour

Children with autism prefer familiar routine and tend to resist change, which they find difficult and unpleasant. They may also have unusual interests, such as in maps or electronic gadgets. They may be very sensitive to light, touch, tastes, smells, and sounds. They may also have odd body movements such as hand-flapping or finger-twiddling.

Any attempt to stop these activities and interests can cause furious protest and distress. When upset, these children may have tantrums, be hyperactive or injure themselves.

Diagnosis

Making the correct diagnosis requires a detailed developmental history, medical and psychological reports, and assessment of the child's social and communication skills and intellectual abilities.

Most parents find that obtaining a correct diagnosis is an important first step. A child's puzzling behaviours become more understandable and it is easier to work out what help they need, now and in the future.

Treatment

Education, with speech and language therapy, offers the most effective way of making sure that a child with autism reaches their full potential.

Children with autism have an increased prevalence of comorbid psychiatric conditions such as ADHD, depression, and anxiety and treating these can be a challenge.

Medication can be effective in combination with behavioural interventions and environmental accommodations in treating comorbid symptoms; however, no medications directly treat the core symptoms of autism.

Further reading

Carr, A. (Ed.) (2000). *'What Works with Children and Adolescents?': A Critical Review of Psychological Interventions with Children, Adolescents and their Families.* London: Brunner-Routledge.

Rutter, M. and Taylor, E. (Eds.) (2002). *Child and Adolescent Psychiatry* (4th edn). London: Blackwell.

Scott, A., Shaw, M., and Joughin, C. (2001). *Finding the Evidence: A Gateway to the Literature in Child and Adolescent Mental Health* (2nd edn). London: Gaskell.

❶ Adolescent-onset psychosis

Definition of psychosis
Psychosis is a disorder in which an individual experiences severe distortions and deviances of cognition and perceptions that they lose sight of the morbid nature of their experiences and their reality testing is impaired.

Signs and symptoms
Positive symptoms
Symptoms of a psychotic illness which affect perception, e.g. hallucinations and delusions.

There are 3 types of positive symptoms:
• Hallucinations
• Delusions
• Confused thinking.

Negative symptoms
• Lack of emotion—the inability to enjoy regular activities (visiting with friends, etc.) as much as before.
• Low energy—the person tends to sit around and sleep much more than normal.
• Lack of interest in life, low motivation.
• Affective flattening—a blank, blunted facial expression or less lively facial movements, flat voice (lack of normal intonations and variance) or physical movements.
• Alogia (difficulty or inability to speak).
• Inappropriate social skills or lack of interest or ability to socialize with other people.
• Inability to make friends or keep friends, or not caring to have friends.
• Social isolation—person spends most of the day alone or only with close family.

Cognitive symptoms of schizophrenia
Cognitive symptoms refer to the difficulties with concentration and memory. These can include:
• Disorganized thinking
• Slow thinking
• Difficulty understanding
• Poor concentration
• Poor memory
• Difficulty expressing thoughts
• Difficulty integrating thoughts, feelings, and behaviour.

Essential elements of the assessment of adolescent-onset psychosis
The essential elements of the assessment of adolescent-onset psychosis are widely agreed and accepted in the UK, North America, and Australia.
These essential elements are:
• *Psychiatric assessment:* a comprehensive diagnostic assessment including an assessment interview with both the patient and the family/carer.
• *Physical examination:* general medical examination to rule out medical causes of psychosis.

Phases of psychosis

- *Prodromal phase*: the prodromal phase is the period of pre-psychotic symptomology and behaviour. The most common prodromal symptoms include magical thinking, unusual perceptual experiences, social isolation, withdrawal, impaired role function, blunted affect, and lack of initiative or energy.
- *Acute phase*: at this stage individuals present with acute delusions, hallucinations, and thought disorder.
- *Recovery phase*: with appropriate treatment the majority of young people successfully recover and return to their normal, everyday lives. Some symptoms of psychosis may still be evident.

Psychiatric formulation

- A diagnosis is made when the prerequisite diagnostic criteria are met and other disorders are ruled out.
- Consideration to the age and developmental level of the young person must be given when considering their explanation of their symptoms.

Treatment

- Low-dose atypical antipsychotic medication if medication is required.
- Psychoeducation for the young person and the family/carers.
- Referral to specialist Early Intervention in Psychosis service.
- In some cases admission to Child and Adolescent Mental Health Services (CAMHS) inpatient provision may be required when there is concern for the safety of the young person or others.

Further reading

Clark, A. (2001). Psychotic disorders. In Gower, S.G. (Ed.) *Adolescent Psychiatry in Clinical Practice*. London: Arnold.

National Early Psychosis Program (1998). *The Australian Clinical Guidelines for Early Psychosis*. Melbourne: University of Melbourne.

National Institute for Health and Clinical Excellence (2009). *Core interventions in the treatment and management of schizophrenia in primary and secondary care (update)* (Clinical Guideline 82). London: NICE.

❶ Eating disorders

Definitions of anorexia nervosa
- Refusal to maintain or achieve body weight at a normal weight for age and height.
- Fear of gaining weight or becoming fat.
- Disturbance in perceptions of body weight or shape.
- Amenorrhoea of at least 3 menstrual cycles.

Definitions of bulimia nervosa
- Binge eating and compensatory behaviours occurring at least twice a week for 3 months.
- Self-induced vomiting, misuse of laxatives, diuretics, enemas, or other medications, fasting or excessive exercise.
- Self-evaluation overly influenced by body shape and weight.

Definitions of eating disorders not otherwise specified
This category includes disorders that do not meet the criteria for a specific eating disorder.

Mortality rates
Eating disorders have the highest mortality rate of any mental illness.

Emergencies can be broken down into 2 broad categories:

Physiological emergencies
These emerge from the effects of starvation or from behaviours utilized to manipulate weight.

Table 7.1 highlights potential risk factors, scores in the concern areas will require regular monitoring and intervention. Score in the red area require urgent medical attention and referral to hospital.

Factors that may escalate into emergency situations if they are not appropriately monitored and managed:
- Electrolyte imbalance: 'refeeding syndrome'. Risk of arrhythmia, cardiac failure, and death.
- Dehydration.
- Vomiting and use of laxatives: gastric or oesophageal ruptures and perforating ulcers.
- Diabetes: abuse of insulin increases risk of hyperglycaemia.

Psychological emergencies
- Severe depression: may lead to non-concordance with treatment.
- Suicide occurs in 2% of the eating-disorder population.
- Lack of insight, motivation, and capacity resulting in non-concordance with treatment.
- Continued refusal to take adequate food and/or fluids.
- Lack of support structures: family, partners.

Table 7.1 Potential risk factors for physiological emergencies

System	Test or investigation	Concern alert
Nutrition	BMI	<14 → <12
	Weight loss/week	>0.5kg → >1.0kg
	Skin breakdown	<0.1cm → >0.2cm
	Purpuric rash	++
Circulation	Systolic BP	<90 → <80
	Diastolic BP	<70 → <60
	Postural drop (sit–stand)	>10 → >20
	Pulse rate	<50 → <40
Musculoskeletal (squat and sit-up tests)	Unable to get up without using arms for balance (yellow)	++
	Unable to get up without using arms as leverage (red)	++
	Unable to sit up without using arms as leverage	++
	Unable to sit up at all	++
Temperature		<35°C → <34.5°C
		<98°F → <97°F
Bone marrow	White cell count	<4.0 → <2.0
	Neutrophil count	<1.5 → <1.0
	Haemoglobin	<11 → <9.0
	Acute haemoglobin drop (MCV and MCH raised—no acute risk)	++
	Platelets	<130 → <110
Salt/water balance	K^+	<3.5 → <3.0
	Na^+	<135 → <130
	Mg^{2+}	0.5–0.7 → <0.5
	PO_4^{2-}	0.5–0.8 → <0.5
	Urea	>7 → >10
Liver	Bilirubin	>20 → >40
	ALP	>110 → >200
	AsT	>40 → >80
	ALT	>45 → >90
	GGT	>45 → >90
Nutrition	Albumin	<35 → <32
	Creatinine kinase	>170 → >250
	Glucose	<3.5 → <2.5
ECG	Pulse rate	<50 → <40
	Corrected QT interval (QTC)	>450msec
	Arrhythmias	++

+ = some signs; ++ = significant signs.

ALP, alkaline phosphatase; ALT, alanine aminotransferase; AST, aspartate aminotransferase; BMI, body mass index; BP, blood pressure; GGT, gamma glutamyl transpeptidase, MCH, mean corpuscular haemoglobin; MCV, mean cell volume.

Management and prevention

- Prevention: regular physical and psychological monitoring, regular weighing, knowing who is doing what (CPA), early intervention.
- Referring to hospital: medical or psychiatric hospital.
- Correction of deficiencies: admission to medical or psychiatric hospital, supplements, via diet, providing education about nutrition.
- Consider assisted feeding: nasogastric, percutaneous endoscopic gastrostomy (PEG).
- Use of the MHA: resistance to interventions, high physiological or psychological risk factors.

Further reading

Birmingham, C.L. and Beumont, P. (2004). *Medical Management of Eating Disorders*. Cambridge: Cambridge University Press.

Palmer, B. (2000). *Helping People with Eating Disorders: A Clinical Guide to Assessment and Treatment*. Chichester: Wiley.

Institute of Psychiatry website: http://www.iop.kcl.ac.uk/sites/edu

Treasure, J. (2004). *A Guide to the Medical Risk Assessment for Eating Disorders*. London: Kings College London, Section of Eating Disorders, Institute of Psychiatry, Eating Disorders Unit, South London and Maudsley NHS Foundation Trust.

❶ Family therapy

Challenges/risks/emergencies

- 'Family therapy' can be seen as a broad term for a range of therapeutic approaches, methods, and techniques for working with families with a wide range of both child- and adult-focused problems.
- Family therapists view difficulties in the context of family relationships/ family interactions and family functioning.
- Family therapists will also consider the wider contextual influences including education, religion, culture, gender, etc.
- Working therapeutically between different time frames, past, present, and future is a core concept of this treatment modality.
- Family therapy work should also consider the influence of the therapists own interpersonal relationships.
- Family therapy focuses on the resourcefulness of clients, moving away from problem-saturated talk, it aims to change patterns of interaction and enable the development of resources and strengthen family communication.
- Therefore family therapy is most frequently not seen as an emergency response to a psychiatric problem but a planned psychotherapy in which a therapeutic contract is reached and goals of the therapy are clear.
- Due to the diversity of family experiences including stepfamily, foster and adoptive family, families with same sex parents, etc. each family will require unique solutions to its problems.
- It is common for the therapist to invite all members of a family and work to engage each person in the process.
- Some areas of family therapy expertise include:
  - Child and adolescent mental health
  - Parenting issues
  - Emotional disorders including anxiety, depression, and grief reaction
  - Anorexia nervosa, bulimia nervosa, and other eating disorders
  - Fostering, adoption and children 'looked after'
  - Drug and alcohol misuse
  - Psychoses.

Risks/emergencies within family therapy

'Emergencies' can arise within the process of the therapy, e.g. it may be necessary to both consider and assess levels of risk during family therapy sessions. However family therapy should not be seen as a treatment to 'fix' 'difficult' families but rather as a collaborative approach with clear aims and goals agreed with the family.

Risk will need to be assessed, e.g. in the following contexts:
- Where there are issues regarding domestic violence.
- Where there are issues regarding mental health, e.g. suicidality.
- Where there are issues regarding child protection/safeguarding for example disclosures of abuse.

The therapist's role is to identify risk and, if appropriate, discuss with the family in a manner that opens up communication to enable planning of risk management strategies. This may include liaison/consultation with other team members and referral to social care. Where possible, the family should be fully involved in the process.

Further reading

Carr, A. (2001). *Family Therapy Concepts, Process and Practice*. Chichester: Wiley.
Burnham, J. (1986). *Family Therapy*. London: Tavistock.
There is also information on the Association of Family Therapy website: ℡ http://www.aft.org.
   co.uk

Emergencies associated with medication

❶ Tardive dyskinesia

Tardive dyskinesia is a movement disorder of late onset which can develop in the course of long-term exposure to antipsychotics. It is characterized by a variety of involuntary movements affecting the muscles of the face, trunk, or limbs.

Symptoms

Symptoms include, most commonly, movements involving the face, eyes, and mouth and may include facial tics, grimacing, tongue protrusion, lip smacking, puckering and pursing, and rapid eye blinking. Movements of the limbs and trunk may also occur such as rocking, twisting, or squirming, foot tapping, ankle movements, and abnormal posture or gait. Symptoms vary considerably even on a daily basis. Severe cases may cause difficulty walking or standing or affect muscles of the larynx or diaphragm leading to difficulty swallowing, speaking, eating, or breathing.

Cause

The mechanism of tardive dyskinesia is unknown. It is believed that prolonged use of medication that blocks dopamine causes hypersensitivity of dopamine receptors and increases the number of D2 receptors in the striated region (involved with motor function) of the brain. This super sensitivity means that stimulation by even a small amount of dopamine may result in muscle contractions and movements. Other agents reported to cause tardive dyskinesia include levodopa, TCAs, and metoclopramide.

Time frame

The onset of symptoms is usually gradual and emerges over a period of months or even years of treatment. Symptoms may last for several months or years after discontinuing the antipsychotic. Most cases are reversible; however, in extremely severe cases, symptoms may be irreversible.

Treatment

Management of tardive dyskinesia should be focused on prevention by using the lowest effective dose of antipsychotic, prescribing atypical antipsychotics first-line, and frequent review of the need for long-term antipsychotic treatment.

If symptoms develop:
- Discontinue any anticholinergic medication as these can exacerbate tardive dyskinesia.
- Attempt to reduce dose of antipsychotic and if possible discontinue treatment. In doing so, the prescribing team must balance the risk of disability against the risk of relapse. Discontinuing the antipsychotic may initially worsen the symptoms of tardive dyskinesia.
- If the patient is prescribed a typical antipsychotic, consider changing to an atypical which poses a significantly lower risk of causing tardive dyskinesia.
- Consider clozapine which has been shown to reduce severity of tardive dyskinesia symptoms.
- Other possible agents include tetrabenazine, vitamin E, and benzodiazepines.

Risk factors

All patients treated with antipsychotics are at risk of developing tardive dyskinesia; however, the risks appear to be greater in the following cases:
- Prolonged exposure to antipsychotics (especially in the elderly).
- Use of high-dose antipsychotics.
- Use of typical antipsychotics.
- Older adults.
- Females.
- History of extrapyramidal adverse effects (e.g. parkinsonism, akathisia) particularly early on in treatment.
- Other possible risk factors include Afro-Caribbean background, affective disorders, negative symptoms of schizophrenia, diabetes mellitus, and alcohol consumption/abuse.

Further reading

American Psychiatric Association (1993). *Tardive dyskinesia: A task force report of the American Psychiatric Association*. Washington, DC: American Psychiatric Association.

Casey, D. and West, E. (1990). Tardive dyskinesia. *Journal of Medicine* **153**: 535–41.

Soares-Weiser, K. and Rathbone, J. (2005). Neuroleptic reduction and/or cessation and neuroleptics as specific treatments for tardive dyskinesia. *Cochrane Database of Systematic Reviews* **3**: CD000459.

Taylor, D., Paton, C., and Kerwin, R. (2007). *Maudsley Prescribing Guidelines* (9th Edition). London: Informa Healthcare.

☼ Oculogyric crisis

Oculogyric crisis is a type of extrapyramidal side effect referred to as an acute dystonic reaction which can be caused by exposure to antipsychotics. It is characterized by a spasmodic movement of the eyeballs into a fixed position, usually upwards.

Symptoms

Initial symptoms may include extreme restlessness, agitation, and a fixed stare. The classic sign is forced deviation of the eyes, usually upwards but sometimes downwards or laterally such that only the whites of the eyes are seen. It is almost always distressing and followed by increased anxiety. Symptoms usually resolve after appropriate treatment.

Cause

Oculogyric crisis is caused by blockade of the D2 receptors in the basal ganglia (striatum). It has been reported with all antipsychotics (both typical and atypical), but also with some other agents (e.g. levodopa, lithium, metoclopramide, benzodiazepines). Other reported causes include Tourette's syndrome, multiple scherosis, head trauma, some types of Parkinson's disease.

Time frame

Symptoms are abrupt in onset and usually appear within hours of starting an antipsychotic (minutes if treatment was parentally). Ninety percent of cases occur within 5 days of exposure to the causal agent(s) (e.g. an antipsychotic).

Treatment

• Immediate treatment with anticholinergic medication is essential. The route of administration depends on severity of symptoms and whether the patient is able to swallow.
• If swallowing reflex is retained, an anticholinergic agent in liquid formulation may be given orally (e.g. procyclidine liquid). Response to treatment is usually 30min.
• If patient is unable to swallow, IV or IM anticholinergic treatment may be necessary. Response to IV treatment is usually within 5min and IM usually about 20min.
• Immediate discontinuation of suspected causal agent(s) is essential.

Risk factors

• Younger patients
• Males
• Neuroleptic-naive patients
• More common with high-potency typical antipsychotics (e.g. haloperidol).

Further reading

Taylor, D., Paton, C., and Kerwin, R. (2007). *Maudsley Prescribing Guidelines* (9th Edition). London: Informa Healthcare.

☢ Anaphylaxis

There is no universally agreed definition of anaphylaxis, but one proposed broad definition is: 'Anaphylaxis is a severe, life-threatening, generalized or systemic hypersensitivity reaction'.

The following three criteria are suggestive of anaphylaxis:
- Sudden onset and rapid progression of symptoms.
- Life-threatening airway and/or breathing and/or circulation problems.
- Skin and/or mucosal changes (flushing, urticaria, angioedema) should be assessed as exposure when using ABCDE approach.

Skin or mucosal changes alone are not a sign of an anaphylactic reaction. Most patients who have skin changes caused by allergy do not go on to develop an anaphylactic reaction.

There can also be gastrointestinal symptoms (e.g. vomiting, abdominal pain, incontinence).

The above airway and/or breathing and/or circulation problems can all alter the patient's neurological status because of decreased brain perfusion. There may be confusion, agitation, and loss of consciousness.

Causes

Anaphylaxis is not predictable, although there are some known agents that are known to cause a higher incidence of anaphylaxis, such as:
- Medicines including antibiotics (e.g. up to 0.05% of patients taking penicillins develop anaphylaxis, of which 5–10% are thought to be fatal), aspirin and other NSAIDs, heparin, parenteral thiamine (e.g. Pabrinex®), and neuromuscular blocking agents.
- Additives and excipients in foods and medicines (such as in depot injections).
- Vaccines (e.g. hepatitis B vaccine).
- Blood products.
- Anaphylaxis is more likely after parenteral administration of medicines.
- Certain foods, including eggs, fish, cows' milk protein, peanuts, and tree nuts.
- Insect stings, in particular wasp and bee stings.

If a patient has an anaphylactic reaction to a certain agent, this should not be given again, as it is likely to induce the same reaction.

Precautions

Resuscitation facilities must always be available when injections associated with special risk are given (e.g. Pabrinex®).

Treatment (also see 📖 Anaphylactic shock, p. 52)

Anaphylactic shock requires prompt treatment of laryngeal oedema, bronchospasm, and hypotension.

When recognizing and treating any acutely medically ill patient, a rational ABCDE approach must be followed, and life-threatening problems treated as they are recognized.
- Airway (A): airway obstruction is an emergency; expert help is needed immediately.

- Breathing (B): immediately assess breathing; vital to diagnose and treat life-threatening conditions, e.g. acute severe bronchospasm.
- Circulation (C): occurs in almost all emergencies; consider hypovolaemia as cause of shock until proved otherwise. Restoration of blood pressure (laying the patient flat and raising the legs, or in the recovery position if unconscious or nauseated and at risk of vomiting).
- Disability (D): common causes of unconsciousness include profound hypoxia, hypercapnia, and cerebral hypoperfusion.
- Exposure (E): to examine the patient properly full exposure of the body is necessary (skin and mucosal changes after anaphylaxis can be subtle). Minimize heat loss and respect patient's dignity.

Cardiopulmonary arrest may follow an anaphylactic reaction; if so, follow the local cardiopulmonary resuscitation policy.

:O: Neuroleptic malignant syndrome

Neuroleptic malignant syndrome (NMS) is a rare, idiosyncratic, and potentially fatal side effect of some drugs, with an estimated incidence of <1%. It can be complex to diagnose as there are commonly many confounding factors, and can be confused with catatonia.

Symptoms

Symptoms include hyperthermia, confusion, fluctuating levels of consciousness, muscle rigidity, and autonomic dysfunction with pallor, tachycardia, labile blood pressure, sweating, and urinary incontinence, and a raised creatine phosphokinase (CPK). There is no recognized spectrum of severity of symptoms.

Cause

As the name suggests it is usually caused by all 'neuroleptics', otherwise known as antipsychotics. It is hypothesized that it is due to over-blockade of the dopaminergic system.

NMS has been reported with all antipsychotics (both typical and atypical), but also with some other agents that affect the dopaminergic system (e.g. drugs used in parkinsonism and related disorders, SSRI antidepressants, venlafaxine, lithium, methylphenidate, metoclopramide, tetrabenazine, and zonisamide).

Because of the low incidence, the diagnostic difficulties, and the varying reports in the literature, it is not possible to confidently differentiate between antipsychotics regarding their associated incidence of NMS.

Time frame

- Symptoms of NMS usually last for 5–7 days after discontinuing the suspected causal agent.
- If an antipsychotic depot formulation has been used, this may be considerably prolonged.

Treatment

- Immediate discontinuation of suspected causal agent(s) is essential (i.e. any antipsychotic).
- A medical opinion should be sought.
- The patient's physical parameters should be closely monitored (blood pressure, pulse, temperature).
- As the syndrome is largely sympathetic overdrive thought to be as a result of dopaminergic antagonism, treatments include dopaminergic agonists such as bromocriptine and dantrolene.
- The patient should be rehydrated.
- Benzodiazepines can be used as short-term sedatives.

Risk factors

- Previous history of NMS
- High-potency typical antipsychotics, e.g. haloperidol
- Recent or rapid dose increases or reductions
- Abrupt withdrawal of anticholinergics, e.g. procyclidine
- Alcoholism

- Hyperthyroidism
- Parkinson's disease
- Learning disability
- Agitation
- Dehydration.

Rechallenging with antipsychotics

- This is inherently associated with a risk of precipitating a repeat episode of NMS, and therefore should be done very cautiously.
- It is recommended that antipsychotics are not re-started for about a week, and only after symptoms of NMS have completely resolved.
- Once the diagnosis of NMS is confirmed, it is usually recommended that an alternative antipsychotic should be started, rather than rechallenging with the suspected causal agent, as there is a high incidence of repeat syndrome occurring on rechallenge.
- Depots (and long-acting injections) should be avoided, and it is recommended to avoid high-potency typical antipsychotics (i.e. haloperidol).
- The chosen antipsychotic should be started at very low doses, and titrated very slowly towards a therapeutic dose. The patient's physical parameters should be closely monitored during this period.

Further reading

British Medical Association and the Royal Pharmaceutical Society of Great Britain (2011, regularly updated). *British National Formulary* (61st Edn). London: BMJ Publishing Group. Available at: ℘ http://www.bnf.org/bnf/.

Taylor, D., Paton, C., and Kerwin, R. (2007). *Maudsley Prescribing Guidelines* (9th Edn.). London: Informa Healthcare.

❶ Rapid tranquillization

Aim

The aim of rapid tranquillization (RT) is to *quickly calm the severely agitated patient, in order to reduce the risk of imminent and serious violence to self or others*—rather than treat the underlying psychiatric condition. The aim is not to induce sleep or unconsciousness. The patient should be sedated but still able to participate in further assessment and treatment.

Principles of RT

Pharmacological treatments

All medication given in the short-term management of disturbed/violent behaviour should be considered as part of rapid tranquillization (including pro re nata [PRN] medication).

- Oral medication should be offered before parenteral treatment is administered.
- The patient must be informed that medication is going to be given, and be given the opportunity to voluntarily accept oral medication at any stage.
- The minimum effective dose should be used.
- Sufficient time should be allowed to elapse for a clinical response between doses.
- IM medication has a faster onset of action.
- Poly-prescribing within a class of medication (e.g. antipsychotics) should be avoided.
- Consider any coexisting medical illnesses and medications, which may impact on dose requirements and potential side effects of medicines for RT.
- Where there is a documented advanced directive/decision, this preference should be adhered to if clinically appropriate.
- In view of the risk of NMS, typical antipsychotics (i.e. haloperidol) should be used with caution in patients previously untreated with antipsychotics, or with an unknown treatment history (see 📖 Neuroleptic malignant syndrome, p. 134).
- The decision to forcibly medicate a patient should be taken jointly by medical and nursing staff.
- Staff involved in physical restraints should be proficient in 'control and restraint' techniques.
- Every effort should be made to provide nursing staff of the same gender as the patient when administering injections in order to ensure safety, privacy, and dignity of the patient.

Commonly used medicines include:

- Oral or IM lorazepam (a benzodiazepine)
- Oral or IM haloperidol (an antipsychotic)
- IM olanzapine (an antipsychotic).

Practical points
- PO and IM medicines should be prescribed separately; the abbreviation 'oral (PO)/intramuscular (IM)' should not be used, as doses may not be bioequivalent.
- Lorazepam should be mixed in a 1:1 ratio; with water for injections before administration.
- *Never* mix drugs in the same syringe.
- Check a patient's allergy and hypersensitivity status before administering any medication (also see ▢ Anaphylaxis; Neuroleptic malignant syndrome; Prescribing, p. 132, 134, 150).

Physical monitoring requirements
In order to ensure the patient's safety, it is essential that the patient's vital signs are regularly monitored and recorded by appropriately trained staff after RT until the patient becomes active again:
- Blood pressure
- Pulse
- Temperature
- Respiratory rate
- Hydration
- Blood oxygen saturation (using pulse oximeters)
- Level of consciousness.

In some circumstances more frequent and intensive monitoring is required.

Risks and complications associated with RT

There are specific risks associated with the different classes of medicines, and specific properties of individual medicines. When medicines are combined, risks may be compounded. All staff prescribing and administering medicines for RT should be familiar with these (refer to the current edition of the *British National Formulary* [BNF] for each specific medicine).

Special populations

- *Older adults:* smaller doses are required. They may be more sensitive to certain side effects. Particular care should be paid to comorbid medical conditions and medication. Both antipsychotics and benzodiazepines may affect mobility and increase the risk of falls. Older adults may have poor muscle perfusion which may produce erratic absorption of IM medicines into the blood stream.
- *Patients under 18 years of age:* smaller doses are required. They may be more sensitive to certain side effects.
- *Pregnancy:* the restraint procedures should be adapted to avoid possible harm to the fetus. Short-acting medicines should be used.

Further reading

British Medical Association and the Royal Pharmaceutical Society of Great Britain (2011, regularly updated). *British National Formulary* (61st Edn.). London: BMJ Publishing Group. Available at: ☍ http://www.bnf.org/bnf/.

National Institute for Health and Clinical Excellence (2005). *Violence: the short-term management of disturbed/violent behaviour in in-patient psychiatric settings and emergency departments* (Clinical Guideline No. 25). London: NICE.

❶ Use of pro re nata or 'as required' medication

PRN medication is prescribed on the PRN section of an inpatient medication chart. These medicines are administered at the nurse's discretion according to the needs of the patient rather than regularly, at a set time each day.

PRN prescription requirements

In addition to general prescription requirements (see 📖 Prescribing, p. 150), PRN prescriptions must also fulfil the following:
- If possible a range of doses should be avoided. If, however, this is necessary the range should be small, e.g. haloperidol 5–10mg.
- Specify the minimum interval between doses/frequency.
- Specify the indication for administration.
- Specify the maximum total daily dose (including any regular prescriptions).
- PO and IM medicines should be prescribed separately, the abbreviation PO/IM should not be used, as doses may not be bioequivalent.

Common PRN prescriptions

The PRN method of prescribing is widely used for treating acute psychotic symptoms, adverse effects of psychotropic medication, or minor physical complaints. Examples include:
- Laxatives for constipation (e.g. senna)
- Anticholinergics for extrapyramidal side effects (e.g. procyclidine)
- Anxiolytics (e.g. lorazepam for anxiety)
- Hypnotics (e.g. temazepam, zopiclone)
- Medications used for RT (e.g. haloperidol, lorazepam)
- Analgesics (e.g. paracetamol, ibuprofen).

Recommendations for PRN prescriptions

All PRN prescriptions should be reviewed at least once a week by the multidisciplinary team. Factors to consider include:
- If the medicine is no longer required, it should be discontinued.
- If repeated administration is required, consider prescribing regularly.
- Repeated administration may indicate severity of a side effect, e.g. frequent use of procyclidine may indicate severe extrapyramidal side effects and may warrant a change in antipsychotic or a reduction in dose.
- The patient's mental state, e.g. repeated need for medication for RT, may warrant an increase/change in antipsychotic.
- Consider alternative non-pharmacological coping strategies before administering PRN medication.

- Particular attention must be observed with the following (especially if the same medication or its constituents are prescribed both PRN and regularly):
  - Timing between doses, e.g. doses of paracetamol must be given at least 4–6h apart.
  - Total maximum daily dose is not exceeded (including any regular prescribed medication).
  - Observe for cumulative adverse effects.
- All PRN prescriptions should be individualized for patients. PRN psychotropics should not be routinely prescribed, medicines should be prescribed based on clinical assessment of the individual patient.

Documentation of administration of PRN medication

- Complete all relevant sections of the inpatient medication chart.
- In the patient's medical notes with details of the medicine administered, date, time, dose, specific symptoms requiring need for administration, and the patient's response to medication. Additionally, documentation should include any non-pharmacological actions taken to prevent PRN psychotropics being administered.

Whilst it is recognized that PRN prescribing is a valuable facility, findings from the recent Prescribing Observatory for Mental Health (POMH-UK) audit of high dose and combination antipsychotics prescribing (2006) confirmed that PRN antipsychotics are major contributors to high doses and polypharmacy.

This section should be read in conjunction with the sections on 📖 Prescribing and 📖 Rapid tranquilization.

Further reading

Chakrabarti, A., Whicher, E.V., Morrison, M., *et al.* (2007). 'As required' medication regimens for seriously mentally ill people in hospital. *Cochrane Database of Systematic Reviews* **3**: CD003441.
POMH-UK website: ℰ http://www.rcpsych.ac.uk/cru/pomh.htm.

❶ Specific medications

Clozapine

Clozapine is indicated for treatment-resistant schizophrenia. It is superior to other antipsychotics in terms of efficacy against positive and negative symptoms, has few/absent extrapyramidal side effects, and reduced rate of suicide in schizophrenia.

Despite its advantages, clozapine can cause some serious, life-threatening adverse effects, notably the risk of agranulocytosis/neutropenia. Consequently it is a mandatory requirement that all patients treated with clozapine in the UK must be registered with an approved clozapine monitoring service to undergo regular blood monitoring of white blood cell, neutrophil, and platelet counts at specified intervals. The majority of cases of neutropenia occur within the first 18 weeks of treatment. This adverse effect is unrelated to the dose prescribed. Other drugs known to be associated with agranulocytosis/neutropenia should not be prescribed in combination with clozapine, e.g. carbamazepine, as this increases the risk.

Clozapine can cause myocarditis and cardiomyopathy. Myocarditis is most common within 6–8 weeks of starting treatment cardiomyopathy usually occurs later. They should be suspected in patients who have persistent tachycardia (rapid heart rate) at rest, arrhythmias (abnormal heart rhythm), palpitations, fever, flu-like symptoms, tiredness, chest pain, ECG changes, any signs of heart failure. Both require prompt discontinuation of clozapine and immediate referral to cardiology.

Seizures can occur with clozapine and are usually related to high- or rapid-dose titration. If a seizure develops, withhold clozapine then restart at a reduced dose and consideration should be given to prescribing sodium valproate.

On very rare occasions, severe increase in blood glucose (hyperglycaemia) has been reported in patients with no prior history of hyperglycaemia. Normalization of glucose levels usually occurs after discontinuation.

Other side effects associated with clozapine include sedation, increased salivation, constipation, tachycardia, nausea, fever, hypertension, hypotension and, over time, weight gain.

Lithium

Lithium is a mood stabilizer widely used for the treatment and prophylaxis of mania, bipolar disorder, and recurrent depression. It has a narrow therapeutic range (see 📖 Therapeutic drug monitoring, p. 158).

Prior to initiation of treatment inform the patient of:
- Baseline tests: ECG, bloods to check TFTs, serum creatinine, U&Es, FBC.
- Need for regular blood tests.
- Symptoms of toxicity and need to report immediately (see 📖 Therapeutic drug monitoring, p. 158).
- Importance to maintain adequate fluid intake and avoid dietary changes that reduce or increase sodium intake.

- Importance to report any conditions leading to salt/water depletion, e.g. vomiting or dieting.
- Importance to carry a lithium treatment card at all times while on treatment.
- Importance of contraception for women of childbearing potential.

Healthcare professionals should be familiar with the common adverse effects of lithium which include gastrointestinal disturbances, fine tremor, hypothyroidism, excessive urination and thirst, as well as the signs of toxicity.

Consequences of interactions with lithium:
- *Increased lithium plasma level:* diuretics, NSAIDs, ACE inhibitors
- *Neurotoxicity:* haloperidol
- *Serotonin syndrome:* SSRIs (see 📖 Serotonin syndrome, p. 156).

Hypnotics

Commonly used hypnotics include the benzodiazepines (e.g. temazepam) and the z-drugs (zopiclone, zolpidem, and zaleplon).

Complications and problems associated with hypnotics include development of tolerance and dependence, rebound insomnia/withdrawal symptoms, and potential for misuse and abuse (see 📖 Discontinuing/ stopping medication, p.154).

General principles of hypnotic use

- First consider non-pharmacological strategies (e.g. good sleep hygiene, sleep diaries).
- Use the lowest effective dose.
- Prescribe PRN and use intermittently to minimize tolerance and dependence.
- Treatment should be time-limited (preferably for only 1 week and no more than 4 weeks).
- Avoid discharging patients from hospital on hypnotics.
- Monitor for rebound insomnia/withdrawal symptoms (e.g. anxiety, nightmares, insomnia, sweating, headache, gastric disturbances).
- Be aware of potential for diversion when prescribing.

Stimulants

Stimulant drugs (e.g. methylphenidate, dexamfetamine) are mainly used for ADHD predominantly in children and adolescents.

Adverse effects include:
- Palpitations
- Nervousness
- Irritability
- Aggression
- Loss of appetite
- Weight loss
- Reduced rate of growth.

Stimulants also have an abuse potential and are therefore legally classed as controlled drugs (CDs).

Further reading

British Medical Association and the Royal Pharmaceutical Society of Great Britain (2011, regularly updated). *British National Formulary* (61st Edn.). London: BMJ Publishing Group. Available at: http://www.bnf.org/bnf/.

National Institute for Health and Clinical Excellence (2004). *Insomnia – newer hypnotic drugs. Zaleplon, zolpidem and zopiclone for the management of insomnia* (Clinical Guideline 77). London: NICE.

❶ Antidepressants and suicide

Suicidal ideas, i.e. thoughts about committing suicide, may be one of the symptoms of severe depression. But the use of antidepressants in the treatment of depression has also been linked with suicidal thoughts and behaviour.

Additionally some of the most commonly used antidepressants, the SSRIs, can cause side effects such as anxiety and associated symptoms (e.g. nervousness), agitation, fatigue, confusion, euphoria, irritability, tremor, psychomotor restlessness/akathisia. Therefore when suicidal ideation or suicidal behaviours are reported during antidepressant therapy, it can be very difficult to distinguish whether these are side effects of the medicines, or whether they may be symptoms of the underlying disease.

Therefore it is good practice for healthcare professionals to always ask patients with depression directly about suicidal ideas and intent.

Monitoring of effects

If it is agreed that an antidepressant should be started, there should be careful monitoring of symptoms, side effects, and suicide risk (particularly in those aged <30 years of age). Patients and carers should be advised to be vigilant for changes in mood, negativity, and hopelessness, signs of akathisia, increased anxiety and agitation, and suicidal ideas, particularly during high-risk periods such as during the first 4 weeks of treatment or when a dose or drug is changed. They should be advised to promptly seek help from a healthcare professional if these are at all distressing.

Choice of antidepressant and supply

Toxicity in overdose should be considered when selecting an antidepressant for patients at significant risk of suicide. The antidepressants with highest risk in overdose are the TCAs (excluding lofepramine), and venlafaxine is more dangerous than the SSRIs. For patients at high risk of suicide, a limited quantity of antidepressants should be prescribed (e.g. 2 weeks' supply).

In children and adolescents

Generally children do not seem to gain the same benefit from antidepressants as adults do. Furthermore in April 2005 the Committee on Human Medicinal Products (CHMP) of the European Medicines Evaluation Agency (EMEA) issued advice on the paediatric use of SSRIs and serotonin noradrenaline reuptake inhibitors (SNRIs) in children, noting that suicide-related behaviour (suicide attempt/self-harm and suicidal thoughts) and hostility (predominantly aggression, oppositional behaviour, and anger) were more frequently observed in clinical trials among children and adolescents treated with these antidepressants, compared with those treated with placebo. Therefore they advised that if antidepressants are prescribed for children and adolescents they should be carefully monitored for the appearance of suicidal behaviour, self-harm, or hostility, particularly at the beginning of treatment.

Currently none of the antidepressants available in the UK are licensed for the treatment of depression in those <18 years old.

Further reading

British Medical Association and the Royal Pharmaceutical Society of Great Britain (2011, regularly updated). *British National Formulary* (61st Edn.). London: BMJ Publishing Group. Available at: ℘ http://www.bnf.org/bnf/.

European Medicines Agency (April 2005). European Medicines Agency finalises review of antidepressants in children and adolescents. [Press release]. Available at: ℘ http://www.ema.europa.eu.

National Institute for Health and Clinical Excellence (2005). *Depression in children and young people: Identification and management in primary, community and secondary care* (Clinical Guideline 28). London: NICE. Available at: ℘ http://www.nice.org.uk/nicemedia/pdf/CG028NICEguideline.pdf.

National Institute for Health and Clinical Excellence (2007). *Depression (amended): Management of depression in primary and secondary care* (Clinical Guideline 23). Available at: ℘ http://www.nice.org.uk/nicemedia/pdf/CG23NICEguidelineamended.pdf.

❶ Pregnancy and lactation

When deciding to use psychotropics in pregnancy or breastfeeding (lactation), decisions should involve the patient, partner, and family. The discussion should include possible risks of exposure to the fetus/infant, weighed against the risks of not treating the mental health disorder. Gestational age, previous response to other treatments, and severity of illness/risk of relapse should all form part of the decision. It is crucial there is clear documentation of all discussions and decisions.

General principles of prescribing in pregnancy and lactation

- When treating any woman of childbearing age with psychotropics, always provide appropriate counselling regarding contraception and the risks of pregnancy, e.g. relapse, risk related with stopping or changing medication, and risk to fetus.
- Some antipsychotics can prohibit menstruation (periods); therefore when changing from one antipsychotic to another consider whether this is likely to affect the menstrual cycle, particularly a return to normal menstruation. If this is likely to be the case, adequate contraceptive measures must be advised in women of childbearing potential.
- Encourage discussion about pregnancy plans.
- Medications that are contraindicated in pregnancy (especially carbamazepine, sodium valproate) should be avoided where possible. If these are prescribed, women should be made fully aware of their teratogenic properties even if not planning pregnancy.
- Medication should only be given if it is clearly necessary.
- Treatment with any medicine should be avoided where possible in the 1st trimester. If this is not feasible, use the lowest effective dose.
- The obstetric team should be informed of any treatment and possible complications.
- Medicines with profiles suggesting lowest risk to the mother and fetus/infant should be chosen.
- Very new drugs are best avoided due to the lack of data on safety in human pregnancy.
- The lowest effective dose should be used balanced with the risk that doses so low may be ineffective in treating the mother's symptoms.
- Monotherapy should be used in preference to combination treatment.
- All prescribing decisions should be regularly reviewed throughout the pregnancy.
- Doses may need adjusting as the pregnancy progresses and physiological changes alter drug handling. Plasma drug level monitoring may be helpful in guiding dosing (see 📖 Therapeutic drug monitoring, p. 158).
- Before a medicine is stopped, the prescribing team should consider:
  - The risk to the fetus/infant and the mother during withdrawal period.
  - The risk of leaving the mother's illness untreated.
- Some psychotropic medicines cross into the breast milk therefore infants who are being breastfed whilst the mother is being treated with psychotropics should be monitored for adverse reactions.
- In breastfeeding, feeds should be timed so as to avoid peak drug levels in milk. Alternatively consider advising the mother to express breast milk to give later.

Current recommendations of drug use

The amount of data for medicine use in pregnancy is constantly increasing, hence Table 8.1 should only be used as a guide and should not be used to influence any clinical decisions. It is important to review the most up-to-date information available when making any clinical decisions.

Table 8.1 Drug use recommendations in pregnancy and lactation

	Pregnancy	Breastfeeding
Antidepressants	Nortriptyline, amitriptyline, imipramine, fluoxetine	Paroxetine, sertraline, nortriptyline, imipramine
Antipsychotics	Chlorpromazine, haloperidol, trifluoperazine	Sulpiride, olanzapine
Benzodiazepines	Regular use is best avoided	Lorazepam
Mood stabilizers	Avoid if possible—consider an antipsychotic	Avoid if possible, valproate if essential. Alternatively consider an antipsychotic
Sedatives	Promethazine	Zolpidem

Timing of exposure

- 1st trimester: exposure of a teratogenic agent/medicine in the first 3 months is more likely to cause structural malformations.
- 2nd/3rd trimester: exposure of a teratogenic agent/medicine after the 1st trimester is more likely to cause growth retardation and neurological damage and have an effect on labour and birth.

Further reading

British Medical Association and the Royal Pharmaceutical Society of Great Britain (2011, regularly updated). *British National Formulary* (61st Edn.). London: BMJ Publishing Group. Available at: http://www.bnf.org/bnf/.

National Institute for Health and Clinical Excellence (2007). *Antenatal and Postnatal Mental Health* (Clinical Guideline 45). London: NICE.

Taylor, D., Paton, C., and Kerwin, R. (2007). *Maudsley Prescribing Guidelines* (9th Edn.). London: Informa Healthcare.

✚ Refusal of medication

If a patient is actively refusing medication, it is essential to talk to the patient directly to establish the reason, with as much explanation as possible.

Patients may refuse medicines for many reasons, for example, because they do not:
• Like its side effects
• Like its effects
• Perceive any benefit
• Like swallowing tablets
• Like its taste
• Swallow tablets
• Like the idea of *having* to take medicines daily
• 'Believe' in conventional medicines, and prefer 'alternative' therapies.

The reason for refusal will guide the management plan. For example alternative medicines can be selected that:
• Don't cause the same troublesome side effect.
• May work more effectively.
• Are available in a different formulation such as a liquid/once-a-day tablet/injection.

There is evidence to suggest that patients are more likely to take medicines if they:
• Perceive that it is of some benefit to them.
• Have a positive relationship with the relevant healthcare professional.

It is also very important to consider the exact medicine that is being refused, its indication, and the potential risks to the patient if it is not taken. Some medicines may cause withdrawal symptoms or discontinuation symptoms if stopped abruptly. If other medicines are refused it may mean that the illness acutely worsens or further complications develop. For example, if an alcoholic patient who is on a chlordiazepoxide detoxification regimen refuses parenteral vitamin B injections, this may become life threatening, and medical help should be sought. Conversely if a patient refuses a hypnotic because he wishes to try sleeping without it, this may be entirely clinically appropriate (see 📖 Discontinuing/stopping medicines, p. 154).

If a patient is refusing prescribed medicines this must be brought to the attention of the prescriber, and the management plan should be discussed with the multidisciplinary team, and documented in medical notes.

When patients are admitted to acute psychiatric wards, nursing staff should carefully observe patients' swallowing of tablets if compliance is questionable. For inpatients held under a section of the MHA, staff should follow the detailed legislation covering the process and documentation required for patients who are not willing to accept their prescribed psychiatric medicines.

Prescribing

Definition

⑦ Prescribing

Definition

To authorize by means of a prescription the supply of any medication.

In the UK, the majority of prescribing remains the remit of doctors, although legislation permits other non-medical staff to prescribe. A prescriber is responsible for the prescription's accuracy and appropriateness for the patient, and legality.

The following are legal requirements for a prescription:
- Clearly, legibly, and indelibly written.
- Dated.
- State the full name and address of the patient (for inpatients the ward/unit and hospital name constitute a temporary address).
- Signed in ink by the prescriber.
- Preferably state the patient's age and the date of birth; this is a legal requirement for prescription-only medicines for children <12 years.

Additionally, the following details should be noted on the prescription:
- Dose and frequency should be stated.
- Formulation should be stated, i.e. tablet, dispersible tables, slow release tablets, liquid, injection.
- Route of administration should be stated.
- Generic names should be used.
- Brand names must be used for specific medicines indicated in the BNF where there is a clinical difference between the brands, e.g. lithium should be prescribed as Priadel®.
- A minimum dose interval should be specified for PRN medicines.
- Avoid decimal points wherever possible; use whole numbers, e.g. 'Digoxin 125 micrograms', not 'Digoxin 0.125mg'.
- Quantities >1g should be written in grams rather than milligrams, e.g. 'Lithium (Priadel®) 1.2g', rather than: 'Lithium (Priadel®) 1200mg'
- Quantities <1g should be written in milligrams rather than grams, e.g. 'Lithium (Priadel®) 800mg', not 'Lithium (Priadel®) 0.8g'.
- Similarly quantities <1mg should be written in micrograms rather than milligrams, e.g. 'Clonazepam 500 micrograms', rather than: 'Clonazepam 0.5mg'.
- It is acceptable to use decimal points to express ranges, e.g. 'Lorazepam 0.5–1mg'.
- 'Micrograms', 'nanograms', and 'units' should not be abbreviated.
- It is unacceptable to use unnecessary abbreviations (e.g. ISMN to mean isosorbide mononitrate).
- Additional requirements are required for PRN prescriptions (see 📖 Use of pro re nata or 'as required' medication, p. 138).

There are additional requirements for 'controlled drugs' ('CDs')—refer to the BNF.

Allergies/hypersensitivities (also see 📖 Anaphylaxis, p. 132)

It is the prescriber's responsibility to check a patient's allergy or hypersensitivity status prior to prescribing any medication. A nurse should also check prior to administration.

Prescriptions for patients detained under the Mental Health Act

For in-patients detained under 'treatment' sections of the MHA, if a copy of Form 38/39 is in place this specifies all prescribed psychiatric medicines that may be given. Any psychiatric medicines that are not detailed on this form cannot be given.

Nurses' responsibilities

- The registered nurse must have knowledge of the patient's assessment, be aware of the patient's treatment plan/pathway, and be satisfied that the prescribed medicine(s) and dose(s) are appropriate for the patient.
- The nurse is responsible for ensuring that the correct medicine is administered, in accordance with the patient's prescription.

Therefore if a nurse is ever unsure about:
- The intention of a prescription (e.g. which formulation of a medicine to be given):
  - *Action:* contact the prescriber to clarify the prescription.
- A medicine (s)he is to administer due to lack of familiarity:
  - *Action:* consult the BNF, other nursing colleagues, a pharmacist, or the prescriber prior to administration.
- The administration process of a medicine (e.g. how to reconstitute a particular injection, or how to use a particular inhaler device):
  - *Action:* consult the manufacturer's leaflets provided with the product, the BNF, a nursing colleague, or a pharmacist.

Action: if ever in doubt about *any* aspect of a prescription—do not administer the medicine, check first.

Remember: the NMC Guidelines for Administration of Medicines.

⚙️ Medication errors

Serious medication errors can harm patients and expose healthcare professionals to civil liability and possibly criminal prosecution. For the first time, the government has set out an aim to reduce the incidence of serious medication errors by 40%.

Role of the National Patient Safety Agency (NPSA)

The Government has set up the NPSA to collect, collate, review, and analyse error reports in order to identify trends and make recommendations to improve safety and reduce risk associated with the use of medicines. This relies on all healthcare professionals reporting all medication errors and near misses so they can feed into the NPSA's national reporting and learning scheme.

The NPSA definition of a *medication error* is any preventable event that may cause or lead to inappropriate medication use or patient harm while the medication is in the control of the healthcare professional, patient, or consumer.

A *near miss* is an error identified with a potential to cause harm.

Common causes of errors

Incidents may be related to any of the steps in the medicine use process: prescribing, dispensing, and administration. Examples are provided in Table 8.2.

Administration errors

- *Frequency:* UK hospital wards have an administration error rate around 5%.
- *Types of errors:* examples include incorrect medicine, incorrect formulation, administration at wrong time, incorrect route, expired medicine administered, 2nd dose administered, incorrect preparation of medicine.
- *Reducing the risk:*
  - Knowledge of the medication including indication, risks, precautions, contraindications, expected outcome.
  - Clarify any uncertainties of the prescription with prescriber or pharmacist prior to administration.
  - If a medicine cannot be administered for whatever reason, notify the prescriber and document details clearly in the medical notes.
  - Check allergy/hypersensitivity status prior to administration.

Apply the '5 rights' prior to administration of any medication

- Right dose
- Right medicine
- Right patient
- Right route
- Right time.

Table 8.2 Common causes of errors and ways to minimize risk

Causes	Possible ways to minimize risk
Prescribing	
<ul><li>Inadequate knowledge of the patient and their clinical condition and allergies/hyper-sensitivities</li><li>Inadequate knowledge of the medicine</li><li>Illegible handwriting or using abbreviations</li><li>Poor medication history</li><li>Calculation errors</li><li>Use of zeros and decimal points</li></ul>	<ul><li>Review long-term repeat prescribing</li><li>Electronic care records and prescribing</li><li>Clear treatment plans shared with all professionals involved in care</li><li>Complex calculations of doses to be double checked</li><li>Avoid unnecessary use of decimal points</li></ul>
Dispensing	
<ul><li>Failure to clarify ambiguous/incomplete/poorly written prescription</li><li>Medicine name confusion</li><li>Similar packaging</li><li>No 2nd check</li></ul>	<ul><li>Formal dispensing and checking procedures</li><li>Staff training and assessment of competency to dispense and check prescriptions</li><li>Additional check of medicines at the point of handing out (with the patient)</li></ul>
Administration	
<ul><li>As a result of errors in the prescribing/dispensing process</li><li>Similar packaging</li><li>Distraction in medication round</li><li>Medicine name confusion</li><li>Confusion between formulations, e.g. modified release preparations</li><li>Omission of doses with no valid reason</li></ul>	<ul><li>Staff training and assessment of competency of staff administering medication</li><li>Double check in certain circumstances, e.g. complex calculations, IV infusions</li><li>Clear medication administration procedures in all settings involved in administering medicines</li><li>Additional check of medicines at the point of administration (with the patient)</li><li>Storing medication safely and neatly to minimize risk of medicine selection errors</li></ul>

Further reading

Department of Health (2004). *Building a Safer NHS for Patients: Improving Medication Safety*. London: DH.

Nursing and Midwifery Council (2008). *NMC Standards for medicines management*. Available on NMC website: ∾ www.nmc-uk.org.

❶ Discontinuing/stopping medicines

Many medicines, particularly those for mental health conditions, should not be stopped suddenly or abruptly, as it may lead to:
- Withdrawal symptoms
- Rebound or discontinuation symptoms
- Relapse of original symptoms of the illness.

Withdrawal symptoms

Some medicines and drugs of misuse are addictive, e.g. opioid drugs (such as heroin and methadone), benzodiazepines, amphetamines (speed), and alcohol. If an addictive substance is stopped abruptly after regular use, it may cause 'withdrawal symptoms'. These may be physical or mental symptoms, the exact symptoms depend on the addictive substance in question, and the seriousness of the symptoms depends on how much of the substance the patient has been taking. Addictive substances usually need to be stopped gradually, and under medical supervision.

For example, common alcohol withdrawal symptoms include:
- Restlessness
- Tremulousness (hands, tongue, or eyelids)
- Fever, with or without infection
- Sweating
- Anxiety
- Nausea/vomiting
- Loss of appetite
- Insomnia
- Tachycardia
- Systolic hypertension
- Psychotic symptoms (visual, auditory, or tactile)
- Generalized seizures.

A substance is addictive if it can cause:
- *Tolerance:* this occurs when the body gets used to the drug or medicine when it is taken regularly, so that you need to take higher doses to have the same effect.
- *Craving:* this is a physical urge, where the body needs the drug or medicine to maintain a desired state or feeling such as euphoria (feeling high), or to avoid an unwanted one such as delirium tremens (the shakes). It can also have a psychological element to it.

Rebound and discontinuation symptoms

If medicines that are not addictive, such as antidepressants, lithium, and antipsychotics, are stopped abruptly, they will not cause the patient to crave the medicine, but the absence may cause other symptoms.

Table 8.3 lists some of the main antidepressant discontinuation/withdrawal symptoms.

Antidepressants should not be stopped suddenly (unless a patient is becoming manic), but should be discontinued gradually, over about 4 weeks.

Some people still experience discontinuation symptoms despite stopping the antidepressant slowly. If symptoms are mild, the patient should be reassured and symptoms monitored. If symptoms are severe, the team should consider reintroducing the antidepressant (or another from the same class with a longer half-life) and reduce more gradually whilst monitoring symptoms.

Table 8.3 Withdrawal/discontinuation effects of common antidepressants

Antidepressant	Withdrawal/discontinuation effects
All antidepressants	'Flu-like' symptoms (chills, muscle aches, sweating, headache, nausea), sleep disturbances including nightmares
TCAs e.g. amitriptyline, dosulepin, imipramine, clomipramine	Excessive salivation, runny nose, diarrhoea, abdominal cramping
SSRIs and **venlafaxine** e.g. sertraline, citalopram, fluoxetine, paroxetine, fluvoxamine	Dizziness, electric shock-like sensations, irritability, crying spells

Relapse of original symptoms of the illness

If a psychotropic medicine is stopped abruptly, the patient's original symptoms may start to return. This doesn't usually happen straight away, it may take 3–6 months after stopping. To avoid this, antidepressants, antipsychotics, and mood stabilizers should usually be gradually reduced before stopping. This is particularly important with some medicines such as lithium and clozapine, where repeated starting and stopping of the agent is thought to lead to a poorer response and prognosis.

Further reading

British Medical Association and the Royal Pharmaceutical Society of Great Britain (2011, regularly updated). *British National Formulary* (61st Edn.). London: BMJ Publishing Group. Available at: ℛ http://www.bnf.org/bnf/.

☼ Serotonin syndrome

Serotonin syndrome is an acute, rare, and potentially life-threatening syndrome. It is pharmacologically predictable, and usually self-limiting if promptly addressed.

Symptoms

Marked neuropsychiatric changes such as:
- Agitation
- Restlessness
- Confusion
- Neuromuscular hyperactivity
- Autonomic instability
- Sweating
- Diarrhoea
- Tremors
- Shivering
- Hyperthermia.

Complications include convulsions, rhabdomyolysis, renal failure, and coagulopathies. Diagnosis is based on Sternbach's criteria; there are no specific laboratory tests to confirm the diagnosis.

Cause

As the name suggests, the syndrome relates to the regulation of serotonin, specifically excess central serotonin activity. It is usually caused by the use of one or more commonly a combination of drugs, which cause excess serotonin to be released, or to remain, in the brain area.

Virtually all antidepressants increase the amount or effect of serotonin in the brain; consequently serotonin syndrome has been reported with numerous antidepressants, as well as with other drugs that affect central serotonin (e.g. buspirone, carbamazepine, tramadol, levodopa, metoclopramide, selegiline, triptans) either alone or in combinations, at therapeutic doses or in overdose.

If not done with due caution, switching between antidepressants can be problematic and can precipitate serotonin syndrome. When switching between antidepressants risks such as discontinuation syndrome (see 📖 Discontinuing/stopping medicines, p. 154), serotonin syndrome, and pharmacokinetic or pharmacodynamic interactions need to be considered. Hence in some cases a total wash-out period or a gap between antidepressants is essential when switching from one antidepressant to another.

Time frame

The onset of symptoms of serotonin syndrome is usually within 24h of a change in serotonergic medicines, and symptoms usually last for about 24h but can persist for longer.

Treatment

- Immediate discontinuation of suspected causal agent(s) is essential (i.e. any antidepressant or other serotonergic agent).
- A medical opinion should be sought.
- The patient's physical parameters should be closely monitored (blood pressure, pulse, temperature).
- The patient should be rehydrated.
- Benzodiazepines can be used to reduce anxiety.
- Removal of the causal agent and supportive measures are usually sufficient; very rarely are more active treatments required.

Risk factors

- Previous history of serotonin syndrome.
- Combination of two potentially serotonergic agents, even at therapeutic doses.

Rechallenging with antidepressants

- This may be done once the patient fully recovers.
- Serotonergic agents should be used alone—not in combination. Starting at a low dose and increasing gradually.

Further reading

Langford, N.J. (2002). Serotonin syndrome. *Adverse Drug Reaction Bulletin* **217**: 831–33.

Sternbach, H. (1991). The serotonin syndrome. *American Journal of Psychiatry* **148**: 705–13.

Taylor, D., Paton, C., and Kerwin, R. (2007). *Maudsley Prescribing Guidelines* (9th Edn.). London: Informa Healthcare.

❶ Therapeutic drug monitoring

Plasma drug level monitoring can be useful to help determine:

- Compliance—the presence absence or the drug in the blood
- Toxicity—for drugs with known toxicity levels, e.g. after an overdose
- Levels may also be used to guide dosing for drugs that have an established target range (i.e. where there is a known relationship between serum levels and therapeutic effect). It is of particular importance if a drug has a narrow therapeutic range.

Drugs with a narrow therapeutic range have a small difference between toxic and therapeutic doses, e.g. lithium and carbamazepine. Minor changes may affect the plasma concentration of the drug (e.g. a drug inter-action, nausea, diarrhoea) and can have significant effects. It is vital that patients on drugs with a narrow therapeutic range have frequent plasma levels and are monitored closely for signs of toxicity.

In the mental health setting, plasma drug monitoring is common with patients on lithium, carbamazepine, and valproate (see Table 8.4).

Interpreting plasma levels

On interpreting plasma levels ensure:

- Ensure the drug is at steady state: plasma levels are only meaningful after steady state has been achieved which is when the rate of drug administration and the rate of drug elimination are equal.
- Ensure the timing of the blood sample is correct: it is essential to know when a plasma sample was obtained in relation to the last dose in order to interpret a level. Incorrect sampling times may lead to misinterpretation of the results.
- Ensure knowledge of the therapeutic range of the drug: plasma levels above the therapeutic range of a drug may indicate toxicity and below the range may indicate subtherapeutic dosing. Ranges differ for different drugs, some are narrower than others. Healthcare professionals need to be familiar with the specific range for the drug as this strongly influences the clinical management of levels.
- Consider the patient's clinical status: if a patient has a plasma level below the therapeutic range but is responding adequately to the treatment, then the dose should not normally be increased. Similarly, if a patient is having intolerable side effects despite the plasma level being within the therapeutic range, consider reducing the dose. Plasma levels above the therapeutic range should usually indicate a dose reduction even if no adverse effects are apparent.

It is essential to know and be aware of the signs of toxicity as well as common side effects.

Table 8.4 Therapeutic drug monitoring of lithium, carbamazepine, and valproate

Drug	Therapeutic range[a]	Sampling time	Time to steady state	Signs of toxicity	Factors increasing plasma level
Lithium	0.4–1.0mmol/L	12h post-dose	5–7 days	Nausea, vomiting, diarrhoea, slurred speech, drowsiness, lethargy, incoordination, coarse tremor, myoclonic jerks, confusion, seizures, coma, death	Sodium/fluid depletion (e.g. vomiting/diarrhoea or dehydration) Impaired renal function Changing the preparation (may alter bioavailability -i.e. absorption of drug) Certain other drug groups e.g. diuretics, NSAIDs, ACE inhibitors
Carbamazepine[b]	8–12mg/L	Pre-dose (trough)	2 weeks	Dizziness, nystagmus (rapid, involuntary eye movements), drowsiness, incoordination, blurred vision, slurred speech, nausea, vomiting	Impaired hepatic function Low albumin Certain drugs, e.g. SSRIs, erythromycin, verapamil
Valproate[b]	50–100mg/L	Pre-dose (trough)	2–3 days	Nausea, vomiting, diarrhoea, abdominal cramps, sedation, tremor, drowsiness, confusion, incoordination, lethargy	Impaired hepatic function Certain drugs, e.g. warfarin, erythromycin, fluoxetine

[a] ranges vary slightly between laboratories.

[b] as mood stabilizers.

Other drugs requiring TDM include gentamicin, vancomycin, digoxin, lamotrigine, and phenytoin.

Further reading

British Medical Association and the Royal Pharmaceutical Society of Great Britain (2011, regularly updated). *British National Formulary* (61st Edn.). London: BMJ Publishing Group. Available at: ℘ http://www.bnf.org/bnf/.

Electronic Medicines Compendium. Available at: ℘ http://www.emc.medicines.org.uk.

Legal frameworks

❶ The Mental Health Act 2007

The detention of patients into mental health services is governed by the Mental Health Act (England and Wales) 2007. The Mental Health Act (MHA) 2007 is essentially an amendment to the MHA 1983. Table 9.1 outlines the main provisions of the Mental Health Act 2007.

Table 9.1 Provisions of the Mental Health Act 2007

Section number and purpose	Maximum duration	Can patient apply to MHRT?	Automatic MHRT hearing?	Can nearest relative apply to MHRT?	Do consent to treatment issues apply?
2 Admission for assessment— application may be made by the nearest relative or an AMHP, and supported by 2 medical recommendations	28 days, not renewable	Within first 14 days	No	No	Yes
3 Admission for treatment— application may be made by a nearest relative or an AMHP, supported by 2 medical recommendations	6mths. May be renewed for 6mths, then annually	Within first 6mths, then in each period	Yes—at 6mths, then every 3 years (yearly if <16) if no application	No	Yes
4 Emergency admission for assessment made by at least 1 medical recommendation	72h. Not renewable but 2nd medical recommen- dation can change to s2	Yes, but only if s4 is converted to s2	No	No	No
5(2) Doctors' or Approved Clinician's holding power	72h. Not renewable	No	No	No	No
5(4) Nurses' holding power	6h. Not renewable, but doctor or Approved Clinician can change to 5(2)	No	No	No	No

(Continued)

Table 9.1 *Continued*

Section number and purpose	Maximum duration	Can patient apply to MHRT?	Automatic MHRT hearing?	Can nearest relative apply to MHRT?	Do consent to treatment issues apply?
7 Reception in guardianship	6mths. May be renewed for 6mths, then yearly	Within first 6mths, then in each period	No	No	No
16 Doctor re-classifies the mental disorder	For the duration of the detention	Within 28 days of being informed	No	No	No
18 Transfer from guardianship to hospital	6mths. May be renewed for 6mths, then annually	Within first 6mths, then in each period	Yes—at 6mths, then every 3 years (yearly if <16) if no application	No	Yes
17 SCT— provisions for people to be discharged from inpatient detention under a CTO	6mths, may be renewed for 6mths, then annually	Within first 6mths, then in each period	Yes—at 6mths then every 3 years	Yes	Yes
25 Restriction of discharge by nearest relative	Variable	No	No	Within 28 days of being informed	
135 Warrant to search for and remove patient	72h. Not renewable	No	No	No	No
136 Police power in public places to remove person to place of safety	72h. Not renewable	No	No	No	No

AMHP, Approved Mental Health Professional; CTO, Community Treatment Order; MHRT, Mental Health Review Tribunal; SCT, Supervised Community Treatment.

Further reading

Department of Health (2008). *Reference Guide to the Mental Health Act 1983*. London: TSO.
Jones, R. (2007). *The Mental Health Act Manual* (11th Edition). London: Sweet and Maxwell.

❶ Mental Health Act 2007: key changes from the Mental Health Act 1983

Definition of a mental disorder

A single definition applies throughout the act; for the purposes of the Act mental disorder is 'Any disorder, or disability of the mind'.

Criteria for detention

People cannot be compulsorily detained unless appropriate medical treatment is available.

Professional roles

The group of professionals able to take on the functions of the Approved Social Worker and Responsible Medical Officer (RMO) is expanded to include Registered Mental Health Nurses, Registered Learning Disability Nurses, Registered Occupational Therapists, and Chartered Psychologists who hold a relevant practising certificate issued by the British Psychological Society and who have undergone further training for these extended powers. These new roles will be called Approved Mental Health Professional (AMHP) and/or Approved Clinician.

Nearest relative

Patients can apply to a county court to displace a nearest relative. The county court can also displace a nearest relative it judges to be unsuitable and civil partners can be named as nearest relatives.

Supervised community treatment (SCT)

It allows for SCT for patients detained in hospital to be discharged on a Community Treatment Order (CTO); the patient remains in detention, but lives in the 'community'.

Electroconvulsive therapy

New safeguards are introduced.

Tribunals

It reduces the period after which hospital managers must refer patients to tribunals if they do not themselves apply.

Advocacy

An appropriate national authority will have a duty to provide support to independent advocates.

Age-appropriate services

Hospital managers must ensure that patients under 18 are treated in a setting suitable for their age.

❶ Section 5(2): doctors' or approved clinicians' holding power

The use of section 5(2)

Section 5(2) grants an approved clinician, i.e. a registered medical practitioner, chartered psychologist, registered mental health or learning disability nurse, occupational therapist or social worker approved by the Secretary of State (England) or Welsh Ministers (Wales)-approved clinician the power to detain a voluntary patient if the clinician believes that the patient needs to be assessed for detention under section 2 or 3. The patient can be detained for up to 72h and it is not renewable.

Issues for the doctor or approved clinician to consider

- The period of detention starts at the moment the doctor or approved clinician furnishes the report to the hospital managers.
- The power cannot be used on a patient attending an outpatient clinic.
- Section 5(2) should only be used if all other attempts to assess the person for detention under the MHA have been exhausted at that point.
- A doctor or approved clinician may nominate a (competent) deputy to exercise their functions under section 5(2).
- Deputies can be nominated by title.
- The hospital managers must let ward staff know who is the nominated deputy.
- A section 5(2) report must not be completed to be used in advance of a voluntary patient wishing to leave.

ⓘ Section 5(4): nurses' holding power

Introduction

The detention of patients into mental health services falls under the auspices of the MHA (England & Wales) 2007. The following is the main provisions of Section 5(4), the nurses' holding powers.

The use of Section 5(4)

Section 5(4) may be used by a Registered Mental Nurse or a Registered Nurse trained in caring for people with learning disabilities to detain an informal patient for a maximum period of 6h, where the detention is necessary for the health and safety of the patient or others, and where it is not possible for the RMO to attend.

Issues for the nurse to consider in using Section 5(4)

- If section 5(4) is invoked, the nurse must endeavour to secure the attendance of the RMO as soon as possible so that the patient can be assessed for detention under another section.
- Under section 5(5) of the MHA the nurse must make a report to management as soon as possible after section 5(4) is invoked.
- If section 5(4) is invoked patients must be informed of their rights under this section as soon as possible thereafter.
- If the RMO detains the patient under 5(2), the 72-h period of this detention starts from the time that the nurse made the report of detention under section 5(4).
- The nurse can make another report for a further 6h detention if the RMO has not arrived before the end of the 6h. However, this is against the spirit of the Act and should be discouraged. It may be possible for the RMO under section 5(3) to nominate someone else to act on his/her behalf.
- Patients detained under section 5(4) cannot be given medication against their will as this section is not covered by Part 4 of the Act governing consent to treatment issues. If might be possible to justify giving a patient medication under section 5(4), using common law powers.
- Section 5(4) can only be used where the patient is an inpatient being treated for a mental disorder. It cannot be used on a patient being treated in a general hospital for a physical illness who becomes mentally ill.

Further reading

Dimond, B.C. and Barker, F.H. (1996). *Mental Health Law for Nurses*. London: Blackwell Science.
Jones, R. (2008). *The Mental Health Act Manual* (11th Edition). London: Sweet and Maxwell.

❶ Sections 135(1) and 135(2)

Introduction
Section 135 is concerned with the forced entry and removal of a person deemed to be suffering from a mental disorder to a place of safety by a police officer on the order of a Justice of the Peace.

Section 135(1)
If a Justice of the Peace deems, from information provided by an AMHP (see 📖 p.164) under oath, that a person believed to be suffering from a mental disorder is unable to care for himself/herself, or is being ill-treated or neglected, the Justice can issue a warrant authorizing any police officer to remove that person to a place of safety so that an application for detention under Part 2 of the MHA can be considered, or other arrangements for the care of said individual can be considered.

If admission to premises where a person thought to be suffering from a mental disorder resides is refused by that person, a Justice can issue a warrant to any police officer to enter the premises, by force if necessary, and remove the person.

A person removed by force and taken to a place of safety may be detained there for up to 72h.

In the execution of a warrant to remove a person by force, a police officer shall be accompanied by an AMHP and a Registered Medical Practitioner.

Section 135(2)
This subsection allows for a warrant to be issued by a Justice of the Peace to a policeman to enter premises, by force if required, to retake a patient who is already detained. This applies to patients on a CTO, those under guardianship, or under the Scottish Mental Health (Care and Treatment) Act 2003, if they have absconded from a place where they are required by law to reside.

People authorized to retake patients under subsection 135(2) are police officers, any officer on the staff of the hospital, any AMHP, any person authorized by the hospital managers, or, in the case of a patient under guardianship, any officer on the staff of the local services authority, or any person authorized by the guardian or local services authority.

Good practices in the use of section 135
Paragraph 10.6, page 73 of the MHA Code of Practice (COP) states: 'When a warrant issued under section 135(2) is being used, it is good practice for the police officer to be accompanied by a person with authority from the managers of the relevant hospital (or local social services authority (LSSA), if applicable) to take the patient into custody and to take or return them to where they ought to be. For patients on supervised community treatment (SCT) it is good practice for this person to be, if possible, a member of the multidisciplinary team responsible for the patient's care'.

Guidance should be available to AMHP on how to obtain warrants (COP, Para. 10.7)

Magistrates should satisfy themselves that a warrant is a last resort and that all other (legal) methods of entry have been exhausted (COP, Para. 10.10)

The AMHP or the Local Social Services Authority should ensure that transport is on hand to take the person to the place of safety (COP, Para. 10.9).

Further reading

Department of Health (2008). *Code of Practice Mental Health Act 1983*. London: TSO.
Jones, R. (2008). *The Mental Health Act Manual* (11th Edition). London: Sweet and Maxwell.

❶ Consent to treatment

Introduction

Sections 57–62 of the MHA are concerned with treatment for which consent is required. Section 64G is concerned with urgent (emergency) treatment.

Section 64G: Emergency treatment for patients lacking capacity or competence

1. In an emergency situation anyone can administer treatment to a patient who they deem to lack capacity to consent to such treatment, but only in the following conditions:
2. The person giving the treatment must believe, reasonably that the person lacks capacity to consent to it, or lacks competence to consent.
3. The treatment must be immediately necessary to save the person's life.
4. The treatment will prevent a serious deterioration of the person's illness and does not have irreversible physical or psychological consequences.
5. The treatment is necessary to prevent the patient causing harm to self or others, represents the minimum level of interference, does not have irreversible physical or psychological consequences, and does not involve significant physical hazard.
6. Treatment may be forced but only to prevent harm, however, the force must be proportionate to the patient suffering harm, and the seriousness of the harm.
7. If the treatment is ECT, or drugs administered as part of ECT, only 3 and 4 apply.
8. Para. 23.25 of the COP states: 'These are the only circumstances in which force may be used to treat SCT patients who object, without recalling them to hospital. This exception is for situations where the patient's interests would be better served by being given urgently needed treatment by force outside hospital rather than being recalled to hospital. This might, for example, be where the situation is so urgent that recall is not realistic, or where taking the patient to hospital would exacerbate their condition, damage their recovery or cause them unnecessary anxiety or suffering. Situations like this should be exceptional'.

Further reading

Department of Health (2008). *Code of Practice Mental Health Act 1983*. London: TSO.
Jones, R. (2008). *The Mental Health Act Manual* (11th Edition). London: Sweet and Maxwell.

❶ Safeguarding vulnerable people

Introduction
The Safeguarding Vulnerable Groups Act (SVGA) was enacted to protect children and vulnerable adults.

Who is a vulnerable adult?
A person aged 18 and over and any of:
- Is in residential accommodation or sheltered housing
- Receives domiciliary care
- Receives any form of healthcare
- Is detained in lawful custody
- Is by virtue of an order of a court under supervision by a person exercising functions for the purposes of Part 1 of the Criminal Justice and Court Services Act 2000 (c. 43)
- Receives a welfare service of a prescribed description
- Receives any service or participates in any activity provided specifically for persons who fall within subsection (9)
- Payments are made to them (or to another on their behalf) in pursuance of arrangements under section 57 of the Health and Social Care Act 2001 (c. 15), or
- Require assistance in the conduct of their affairs.

Key features of the SVGA
- An Independent Barring Board (IBB) will decide whether a person should be barred from working with vulnerable people.
- People barred by the IBB can appeal the decision.
- Two types of activity are defined within the SVGA: regulated activity refers to people who will be working at the frontline with direct access to vulnerable people. Controlled activity gives some access to vulnerable people, but not that defined by regulated activity
- A person who seeks or engages in regulated activity with a vulnerable person or groups, when they are barred, or have not been checked, is committing an offence
- Regulated activity providers (RAPs) are companies that provide regulated activity. They must not employ people to work with children and vulnerable adults that they know are barred from working with such people.
- RAPs who wish to employ people to work with vulnerable children or adults must ensure through Criminal Records Bureau checks that such people are not barred from so doing.

Further reading
Department of Constitutional Affairs (2006). *Safeguarding Vulnerable Groups Act 2006*. London: DCA.

❶ Mental Capacity Act 2005

Introduction

The Mental Capacity Act (MCA) came into force on 1 April 2007. The Act is designed to provide legislation to protect people who may lack capacity to make their own decisions, clarifies who can take these decisions, when they can take them, and how to exercise these functions if required. The Act also people to make advance decisions (directives) to plan for when they make lack capacity. The Act does not apply to people aged <16.

The scope of the MCA

The MCA covers the key decisions about people's property and affairs, health and social care treatment, and decisions about personal care in the event that they lack capacity to make their own decisions.

The principles of the MCA

Five principles underpin the operation the execution of the MCA:
1. A person must be assumed to have capacity unless it is established that he lacks capacity.
2. A person is not to be treated as unable to make a decision unless all practicable steps to help him to do so have been taken without success.
3. A person is not to be treated as unable to make a decision merely because he makes an unwise decision.
4. An act done or decision made, under this Act for or on behalf of a person who lacks capacity must be done, or made, in his best interests.
5. Before the act is done, or the decision is made, regard must be had to whether the purpose for which it is needed can be as effectively achieved in a way that is less restrictive of the person's rights and freedom of action.

Definition of lack of capacity within the MCA

- Inability to make a decision regarding a particular matter due to temporary or permanent impairment of, or disturbance in the functioning of the mind or brain.
- A lack of capacity cannot be established simply by reference to a person's age, appearance, or behaviour, which might lead others to make unwarranted assumptions about capacity.
- Whether a person lacks capacity within the meaning of the MCA must be decided on the balance of probabilities.

Definition of inability to make decisions within the MCA

- Inability to understand information relevant to the decision.
- Inability to retain information.
- Inability to use or weigh information as part of the process of making the Decision.
- Inability to communicate the decision by whatever means.

If a person is able to understand information in a way that is appropriate to his/her situation, e.g. using simple language, visual aids, they are not judged as unable to understand the information, even if they can retain the information for only a short period.

Definition of best interests within the MCA

Section 4 of the MCA defines best interests. A person appointed to determine the best interests of another must, as far as it is possible to do so:

- Take account of that person's past and present wishes, especially if these have been written, such as in an advance directive when the person had capacity.
- Consider the person's beliefs and values that might have influenced their decision.
- Consider whether the person might regain capacity, and when this might be.
- Take into account all relevant circumstances.
- Encourage the person to participate in the decision-making.
- Take account of, or consult the views of others who know the person, e.g. carers, lasting power of attorney or anyone appointed by a court.

Further reading

Bartlett, P. and Sandland, R. (2007). *Mental Health Law: policy and practice* (3rd Edition). Oxford: Oxford University Press.
Department for Constitutional Affairs (2005). *The Mental Capacity Act 2005*. London: DCA.

❶ Mental Health (Care and Treatment) (Scotland) Act 2003

Table 9.2 Mental Health (Care and Treatment) (Scotland) Act 2003

Section/Part	Duration	Mental Welfare Commission/ Mental Health Tribunal	Appeal	Consent
36 Emergency detention in hospital	72h	MWC informed if MHO consent not obtained	No. Can be revoked by Approved Medical Practitioner	MHO, where practicable
44 Short-term detention in hospital	28 days, can be extended by 3 days prior to CTO	MWC/ MHT to be informed within 7 days	Patient/named person can apply to Tribunal for revocation of certificate	MHO. Named person to be informed
299 Nurse's holding power	2h. Can be extended by 1h to allow examination to be carried out	MWC to be informed in writing	No	No
Part 7 CTO treatment enforced either in hospital or community setting	6mths, followed by 6mths, then 12-mthly	Tribunal makes decision on application	At time of Tribunal hearing and after 3 months	No
Interim CTO when further assessment required prior to applying CTO	28 days, further 28 days, maximum 56 days	Tribunal makes decision	At time of Tribunal hearing	No
112 Detention in event of failure to attend for treatment under CTO	6h	HO consulted	No	MHO consent required

(Continued)

Table 9.2 *Continued*

Section/Part	Duration	Mental Welfare Commission/ Mental Health Tribunal	Appeal	Consent
130 Assessment of mentally disordered offenders	28 days	RMO must report to court before end of 28 days	No	No
133 Compulsion order for mentally disordered offenders	6mths but under regular review by RMO	RMO must report to court if order no longer appropriate	No	No
134 Detention of acquitted persons for assessment	6h	MWC to be informed within 7 days	No	No

CTO, Community Treatment Order; MHT, Mental Health Tribunal; MWC, Mental Welfare Commission.

Index